How to Save Your Brain

Your Basic Toolkit for Beating Memory Loss and "Mind Fog" from Age 38 to 88!

By Weldon Reed

How to Save Your Brain
Your Basic Toolkit for Beating Memory Loss and "Mind Fog" from Age 38 to 88!

Published by Online Publishing & Marketing, LLC

IMPORTANT CAUTION:

By reading this special report you are demonstrating an interest in maintaining good and vigorous health. This report suggests ways you can do that, but – as with anything in medicine – there are no guarantees.

The author, editors and publishers of this report are not doctors or professional health caregivers. The information offered in the report is not meant to replace the attention or advice of physicians or other healthcare professionals. Nothing contained in this report is meant to be personal medical advice for any particular individual.

Every reader who needs treatment for a disease or health condition should first get the advice of a qualified health care professional.

The author, editors and publishers believe the information in the report is accurate, but its accuracy cannot be guaranteed. They are not responsible for any adverse effects or results from the use of any of the suggestions described in the report. As with any health treatment or lifestyle change, results of the treatments described in this report will vary from one person to another.

Contents

Introduction

How to Save Your Brain

Grocery lists… names of family members and friends… memorable vacations… directions to your favorite restaurants – all these things are neatly filed away into the various compartments of your brain ready to be recalled – *within seconds* – whenever you need them.

The brain is truly an amazing creation, as proved by the speed at which it operates to meet the demands of all the situations you encounter. That being said, you have to make a constant and dedicated effort to keep your brain healthy if you want to think – and live – at the highest level of function you can.

There are millions and millions of intricate connections in the brain. Every time you have a new thought or recall a memory you create a new connection in your brain. The health of these intricate connections is the foundation of a healthy and strong mind. Any type of interruption in their microscopic functions can potentially spark the beginning of early brain decay, putting you at greater risk for a host of problems – even diseases.

Poor brain function is something you must prevent at all cost if you want to ensure your brain is able to meet the daily demands of your life.

Sadly, there are a variety of different factors that can impede or slow down the intricate connections in your brain without your even realizing it. When this starts to happen, your risk for memory problems and brain diseases goes up significantly.

That's why it's important to identify any potential hazards that can be subtly attacking your brain before the damage leaves permanent scars…

Chapter One

Four Things You're Probably Doing Right Now That Shrink Your Brain

Heed the warning signs now – and stop making these common mistakes!

What makes the brain so unique compared to any other organ is that it's able to use other parts of the body to warn you when you've got a health problem.

Every single function in the body can have a direct connection to how well your brain is working. Most people wait till they start noticing an actual decline in their memory and their thinking ability before they pay attention to their brain health. But most likely you'll see other problems in your body *before* you see cognitive decline.

"Cognitive decline" is a fancy word for *brain loss*. You know brain loss has begun when you. . .

- Walk into a room and can't remember why you went there. . .

- Can't remember where you put your keys. . .

- Can't remember a friend's name. . .

- Can't remember a word, or a date, or a fact you know very well. . .and then it comes to you an hour later. . .

Your doctor may tell you that losing your memory is just a normal part of aging. Don't believe it! In reality it means **your brain is literally shrinking**. And it's not normal. It's an early sign of disease.

What's more, you can slow it down, stop it and even *reverse* it!

Every day, you're probably doing four things that shrink your brain. These mistakes cause you to lose not only your memory but also your ability to think fast and make decisions. I know you're probably making these four brain-killing mistakes because almost EVERYBODY makes them.

And it's easy to know you're making these four mistakes because *your body tells you.*

Don't wait till things get really bad and you can't remember the names and faces of those you love – or even how to eat or go to the bathroom! Yes, that's what happens when you have Alzheimer's and other types of dementia.

But you can spot brain loss early and stop it, because your body lets you know you've got a brain problem way ahead of time. The brain uses other areas of your body to signal that something is wrong. If you learn to pay attention to these common symptoms, you can help avoid the risk of brain decay, age-related memory loss, foggy thinking and degenerative diseases like Alzheimer's.

Instead, you can hold on to your foolproof memory and "wow" your friends and family with your mental fitness for years to come.

These are the four surprising factors that may be symptoms of poor brain health – and what to do about them…

The hidden link between chronic back pain and memory loss...

You may think waking up in the morning with back pain is just one of the hazards of getting older. People tend to look at constant aches as normal aging.

Big mistake.

It's true that the older you are, the more likely you are to suffer from back, muscle and joint pain. But that does NOT mean you should accept them as "normal." They aren't. They're a symptom of bad health and can be corrected if you take a few easy steps.

What's more, there's a little-known connection between back pain and brain health. Researchers have found that people who suffer from chronic back pain also report various degrees of memory loss. The two medical problems share a common cause.

Under normal circumstances, if a person reports both back pain and memory loss to a doctor, the doctor's response will be to treat the two problems separately. Of course, the majority of doctors might think memory loss means the person may be at risk for Alzheimer's disease or dementia. But most doctors will see no reason to connect memory loss to back pain.

However, scientists have found chronic back pain and Alzheimer's disease have something in common: I'm talking about **chronic inflammation**.

As you may know, inflammation is the body's natural response when there is an injury or potentially dangerous threat to health. It's a result of the immune system's response to a cut or an infection, for example. The activity produced by inflammation allows the body to heal an injury or remove harmful bacteria, toxins, viruses and fungi that can threaten overall health. The pain, swelling and redness you feel are your body killing off germs.

Chronic inflammation is something different. It doesn't end when the short-term threat (like a cut or infection) ends. It goes on and on, causing substantial long-term damage and, in some cases, even death. Arthritis is a typical example of long-term, chronic inflammation. So is heart disease.

You should assume this if you suffer from chronic pain

Please know this: if you've got chronic pain, most likely it's not just your bones and joints that are inflamed. Other body parts will suffer from inflammation, too – including your brain.

People suffering from chronic back pain experience frequent bouts of inflammation. Victims will often take over-the-counter pain relievers. And when pain symptoms become too hard to manage, a doctor may prescribe anti-inflammatory medications.

How does chronic inflammation affect the brain? This is how: What should be a normal, healthy immune response turns on you and becomes destructive.

Over time, chronic inflammation begins to attack and destroy a wide range of body parts: individual cells… muscles… bones… and your most vital organs. This destruction can go undetected for years.

Usually you don't feel or recognize chronic inflammation until more serious health problems develop and the full effect starts to become obvious. But there's good news: **You can watch your pain disappear – and get rid of the threat to your brain at the same time.**

In just a minute, I'm going to tell you the four best natural ways to control inflammation.

Inflammation targets precious brain cells and

What Causes Vitamin D Deficiency

By eliminating common risk factors associated with vitamin D deficiency, you can help ensure your brain and the rest of your body receive all the benefits of this remarkable nutrient.

The most common causes of vitamin D deficiency are:

- **Lack of vitamin D in your daily diet** – Meeting the recommended levels of vitamin D has to be a long-term commitment. If your diet does not include foods that contain adequate amounts of vitamin D, the risk for deficiency will be high. Natural food sources for vitamin D come from animal-based products such as fish oil, so it is important to know a vegetarian diet can trigger vitamin D deficiency.

- **Poor kidney function** – The kidneys are responsible for converting vitamin D into its active form, but aging causes kidney function to slow down. This is one reason why elderly people often lack adequate levels of vitamin D.

- **Limited sunlight exposure** – Cases of Alzheimer's disease are generally higher in northern climates verses tropical ones. People who are exposed to more sunlight will enjoy higher levels of vitamin D because, when skin is exposed to sunlight, it produces the vitamin naturally. Staying indoors… constantly covering your skin… and living in northern latitudes are factors that limit your exposure to sunlight.

- **Pigmentation** – People who are dark skinned have the highest risk of vitamin D deficiency. Studies show this risk is even higher for seniors with dark skin. The melanin in the skin determines how much pigmentation a person has. The more melanin – the darker the skin. The darker the skin – the harder it is for the skin to respond to sunlight and make vitamin D.

http://www.webmd.com/diet/vitamin-d-deficiency

breaks down the integrity of brain tissue. Memory and other cognitive abilities pay a high price for this loss of brain cells. The risk of developing diseases like Alzheimer's and dementia soars.

So if you suffer from back pain, assume your other tissues and organs are under attack, even if you can't feel it yet. Take steps to protect yourself. Don't go on allowing inflammation to silently attack your brain. Get to the root cause and put out the fire before you run the risk of losing your mind.

BUT. . .anti-inflammatory medications – so-called NSAID drugs – are not the answer.

It's important to note using these drugs to treat inflammation can pose another potential threat to brain health.

Will an Advil a day keep Alzheimer's away?

There have been many cases where people suffering from chronic back pain have been prescribed pain medications or have started taking over-the-counter pain-killers like ibuprofen (the ingredient in Advil) or, of course, aspirin. They do indeed experience pain relief and may even notice improvements in memory. Long-term use of ibuprofen, for example, is actually associated with a slowing down in the progress of Alzheimer's symptoms.

But an important study indicates the improvement doesn't last. After taking these medications for two years, participants reported their Alzheimer's symptoms actually got worse. That's because anti-inflammatory drugs cause serious soft tissue damage – and you guessed it – the brain is composed of soft tissue.

You need to fight inflammation with more natural – and safer – alternatives that don't destroy delicate brain tissue. But it should be noted that brain damage is not the most common side effect of NSAIDs. The most common side effect is **intestinal bleeding and damage to the intestinal tract**.

Many people who take anti-inflammatory drugs develop ulcers – some very quickly, some after a year or two. And a substantial number of these people actually die – not from whatever was causing their inflammation, but from the drug they took to relieve it!

When you take them long term, every day, drugs like aspirin and ibuprofen are extremely dangerous. They kill thousands of people a year, and cause thousands more to become seriously ill.

The *American Journal of Medicine* says 107,000 people a year are hospitalized because of gastro-intestinal side effects of NSAID drugs, and *at least* 16,500 die. The prestigious *New England Journal of Medicine* said NSAIDs would be the 15th leading cause of death in the United States if the figures were tallied separately.

Turn instead to the many <u>natural</u> anti-inflammatory nutrients available in whole foods and in supplements. They can help you reduce chronic inflammation gently, relieve your pain, and at the same time lower your risk for Alzheimer's disease and many other conditions related to chronic inflammation, including diabetes, cancer and heart disease.

The four best natural anti-inflammatories

If you're looking for fast, long-lasting relief from inflammation – **proteolytic enzymes** are an absolute must! Proteolytic enzymes are those that help you digest proteins. They're also called **proteases** (pronounced pro-tee-ā-zes). Studies show they're the most powerful natural resource available to fight inflammation.

Your body actually makes its own proteolytic enzymes, and they're its first line of defense against painful inflammation. The enzymes go even further – they work to reverse the damage caused by inflammation. They have the potential to help slow down the progress of Alzheimer's and dementia as well as heart and artery disease, diabetes, arthritis and even cancer.

Probably the best news about proteolytic enzymes is that they're free of side effects and deliver better anti-inflammatory benefits than conventional drugs. A wide variety of enzymes is available in any good supplement store.

If you currently suffer from chronic back pain or other symptoms of chronic inflammation, start supplementing with proteolytic enzymes as soon as possible to safely relieve your symptoms and preserve brain health. Enzymes aren't drugs – they're natural, healthy foods. Many people get very quick pain relief, and almost everyone sees results if they take enzymes long term (as you should).

Of course, enzymes are not the only natural anti-inflammatories. The spice **turmeric** is also highly effective. You can take the active ingredient in turmeric, called **curcumin**, as a supplement.

Another excellent way to reduce inflammation is **omega-3 oils**, including fish oils and flaxseed oil. As you may know, omega-3 oils also support heart and artery health. Omega-3 oils are among the most widely-prescribed natural food supplements in the world.

Evening primrose oil contains an omega-3 oil not present in fish and flaxseed oil. It is an extremely valuable anti-inflammatory. Research indicates the combination of evening primrose oil with either fish oil or flaxseed oil packs greater anti-inflammatory power than any one of them by itself.

A few months on these safe, natural foods will go a long way toward putting out the fire in your body, including the one that's scorching your brain.

Now let's go to the second warning sign of brain loss. It's a big mistake to let this slide without doing something about it. . .

An upset tummy can mean an upset brain...

Do you suffer from chronic digestive problems? Have you noticed any abnormal changes in your digestion as you've gotten older? Would you say the overall health of your digestive tract is good? For tens of millions of people, the answer is no.

Millions of people suffer from ulcers, acid reflux or GERD, constipation, gas, diarrhea – and even parasites and infections.

It might surprise you to know that what happens in the stomach can give you insight into the health of your brain, because there's a powerful connection between the stomach and the brain. Every time you experience a feeling of "butterflies" or a "sinking feeling" in your gut – it means your brain is using your stomach to tell you something.

The health of the stomach – especially the state of your intestinal flora or "friendly bacteria" – can be a valuable symptom if you want to know how well your brain is functioning.

The bacteria in your intestine comprise 100 trillion organisms made up of roughly 500 different species (although few people have all 500). In fact, you have more bacteria in your digestive tract than you have cells in your entire body. The bacteria are smaller than human cells, so they don't make up as much total weight as the rest of your body.

The bacteria in the digestive tract are responsible for:

• Absorbing calcium… magnesium… and zinc

• Boosting immune function

• Breaking down and absorbing food

• Producing B vitamins and vitamin K

So how do intestinal flora specifically relate to the health of your brain and memory?

Intestinal flora contain both good bacteria and bad bacteria. The two types compete with each other, and a balance has to be strictly maintained between them, if you want to enjoy good health. There's no need to completely eliminate bad bacteria – it's probably impossible. But healthy levels of good bacteria are needed to keep the bad ones in check.

Intestinal bacteria help determine how well food is digested. If you're not digesting your food properly, nutrients won't be successfully transported to the brain to keep it well nourished.

When bad bacteria overpower good bacteria – a condition called dysbiosis – it creates a vast quantity of toxic byproducts called lipopolysaccharides. These are a nightmare for the brain.

These toxins negatively affect the brain by:

- Decreasing dopamine and serotonin levels; these neurotransmitters are essential to good health

- Increasing oxidative (free radical) damage

- Inflicting serious damage to the hippocampus – the area of the brain that houses memory activity

- Raising stress hormone levels

- Triggering inflammation

If you let them run wild, toxic lipopolysaccharides can destroy your brain health and take a dreadful toll on your cognitive abilities – your ability to remember things and think clearly .

These common prescription drugs can upset your digestion AND rob your memory

A number of factors can contribute to an imbalance or deficiency in intestinal bacteria. Aging, stress, pesticides from foods and environmental pollutants are just some of the many factors linked to an overgrowth of bad strains of bacteria in your gut.

However, antibiotics are probably the biggest threat to your intestinal flora. Taking prescription antibiotics can do extremely serious long-term damage to the balance of bacteria in the intestinal tract.

Because antibiotics are prescribed so frequently – often for illnesses like colds and flu, where they do no good – nearly every American has taken these drugs at some time or other. Many of us have taken multiple courses of antibiotics, and some of us have taken them for months or years at a time. *In terms of digestive health, this has been a national disaster*.

Taking antibiotics wipes out both the good and bad bacteria inside the digestive tract. The resulting bacterial imbalance or dysbiosis is marked by symptoms such as diarrhea… abdominal cramps… nausea… and even yeast infections.

If you suffer from almost ANY gastrointestinal problem, the antibiotics you've taken are a prime suspect, even if you took them years ago.

Fight Dementia with Vitamin C and Beta-carotene

The Journal of Alzheimer's Disease recently published a study that supported the need to supplement with vitamin C and beta-carotene if you want to lower your risk of dementia.

The study found that senior adults who suffer from dementia had significantly lower levels of both vitamin C and beta-carotene in their blood, compared to the blood samples of healthy seniors with normal cognitive activity.

The antioxidant capabilities of these two nutrients provide superior protection against dementia-related neurodegeneration than all other nutrients that were studied.

Clearly then, vitamin C and beta-carotene need to be in your nutrient arsenal to lower your risk for dementia.

http://medicalxpress.com/news/2012-09-vitamin-beta-carotene-dementia.html

To prevent the kind of environment where bad bacteria flourish, it's important to counteract the negative effects of antibiotics by supplementing with healthy probiotics. Probiotics are simply food supplements that contain live bacteria and yeast cultures proven to promote a healthy gut.

Fermented foods like yogurt can also provide probiotic cultures, but many brands of store-bought yogurt don't contain many live cultures. It's pretty hard to obtain the live cultures you need from foods. That's why probiotic pills or capsules are recommended.

Look for a probiotic supplement that contains at least 10 to 20 billion active microorganisms, made up of multiple different strains of healthy or "good" bacteria. Some probiotic supplements contain 15 or 16 different species of bacteria, and that's highly desirable. Generally speaking, probiotic supplements need to be refrigerated – because they're made up of fragile living cells. Brands that haven't been refrigerated are suspect.

Two common, healthy bacteria strains to look for are lactobacilli and bifidobacteria. They'll be listed on the label of a probiotic product. These and other healthy strains help restore the balance of good bacteria to intestinal flora and prevent damage to your brain. Read the label to see what strains of bacteria the product contains, and how many total organisms. Generally, the more the better. The best brands contain as many as 100 million bacteria per serving.

There's no toxicity associated with healthy probiotic supplements and you can safely take 100 million bacteria a day, or even more, until normal bowel function has been restored. Probiotic supplements are actually a proven medical treatment for diarrhea.

What's good for your gut is good for your brain

How do you know when your bowel function is back to normal? That's easy. If you suffer from either diarrhea OR constipation, you don't have normal bowel function. Contrary to what some "experts" may tell you, these conditions signify serious bad health. You should have *at least* one bowel movement per day. It should be soft and easy (but not watery) and it should come out pretty fast, with no straining.

Here's something else that's important: You need to supplement with probiotics for life, because – unlike your own intestinal bacteria, which you developed as a baby and toddler – the ones you introduce into your body by supplements die out after a time and have to be constantly replenished. If antibiotics have essentially wiped out your own "native" intestinal flora, the ones you developed as a baby, then you need to remain on probiotic supplements for good.

Keeping the digestive tract healthy and in balance will help make sure the brain does not become malnourished or exposed to harmful toxins. These toxins not only decrease brain activity but damage your general health as well.

Now for the third common mistake that can shrink your brain. . .

If you don't brush and floss you might lose your mind

Recent studies have found when you brush and floss your teeth you do much more than give yourself an attractive smile. You also protect your brain!

A team of British dentists and psychiatrists conducted a unique study and determined a clear connection between oral hygiene and the ability to think straight…

In this study, researchers examined the oral hygiene of thousands of people ranging in age from 20 to 59. They discovered that people with gingivitis and periodontal (gum) disease had poor cognitive activity during their adult life that continued into their later years.

The most likely reason is that gum disease is related to – you guessed it – inflammation. The bacteria that inflame the gums may be systemic – that is, they may affect your whole body and cause inflammation from head to toe.

Gum disease has already been linked to heart and artery disease and to cancer as well. So it's no surprise it damages the brain. Infected gums affect the whole body. They're a serious burden on your overall health and wellbeing.

Don't let your oral health fall by the wayside. Brush and floss your teeth for several minutes at least once a day, and two or three times if you can manage it.

And here's the fourth common mistake that can shrink your brain. . .

You can help restore your brain with something that's *easy*, *pleasant* and *free*!

Sleep is a powerful way to restore and revitalize a sluggish brain. First and foremost, a good night's sleep allows the mind and body to relax and get a break from the constant work they have to do when you're awake.

So it seems weird that 43% of Americans are so tired during the day it interferes with their normal, daily activities. And one-third admit they need eight hours a night, but their average sleep time is less than seven.

There's more at stake than just feeling a little drowsy after lunch. Severe cognitive impairment can result if you short-change the brain on quality, restful sleep. Time and time again, research has demonstrated a consistent link between sleep and optimum mental ability.

Concentration… physical performance… memory… and mental reaction time are just a few cognitive abilities that depend (in part) on the amount of good sleep you receive each night.

Sleep poorly, lose your mind

The Mayo Clinic reported that mild cognitive impairment – MCI – can be caused by various sleeping disorders known for disrupting sleep patterns. MCI is the early stage of Alzheimer's and other forms of dementia.

Other studies have revealed an even more serious fact: Lack of sleep may actually kill brain cells. It goes without saying, this opens you up to a higher risk of cognitive difficulties and poor brain health.

It's often been observed that poor sleep is one of the side effects of Alzheimer's disease. The victims don't sleep well. However, more in-depth scientific studies are actually showing this is not the whole picture.

According to this new research, scientists are now leaning toward the view that the cause and effect also go the other way around: Alzheimer's may be a side effect of poor sleep! In other words, being sleep-deprived may increase your risk of Alzheimer's disease.

According to the results of a study conducted at Washington University School of Medicine, people who wake up frequently during the night have much higher concentrations of amyloid plaque in their brains. A large amount of amyloid plaque is the defining sign of Alzheimer's.

When this plaque clumps together and builds up in the brain, neurons die. What follows is an increase in both the frequency and severity of symptoms associated with brain diseases like Alzheimer's.

It happened to these lab animals and it could happen to you

Animal studies brought the connection between Alzheimer's and sleep to light when a team of experts took mice genetically predisposed to Alzheimer's plaque build-up and altered their sleeping patterns for three weeks.

The sleep-deprived mice – which were only allowed to sleep four hours a day – had more plaque in their brains than the well-rested mice.

Scientists also found the protein level in amyloid plaque increased in mice during wakefulness and decreased while they slept, supporting the theory that sleep is essential in reducing amyloid plaque levels. And it's not only true of old animals. This same fluctuation in protein levels was also seen in samples taken from young, healthy adult animals. They experienced the positive benefits of sleep in regulating this potentially dangerous protein.

These study results provide an important insight into the relationship between sleep and brain health. **The mouse study in particular found a direct link between disrupted sleep and**

the growth of brain plaques – the one physical process that scientists know for sure is a marker for Alzheimer's disease.

An animal study isn't conclusive. Human studies are needed. But there's enough other evidence to indicate without a doubt that lack of sleep damages your brain.

Look at it this way: Sleep is like a "drug" that brings your brain back to health. But you can "prescribe" it to yourself and it doesn't cost a penny. It's more powerful than any of the prescription drugs now available for Alzheimer's. At best, the drugs slow down memory loss a little bit. By comparison, the effects of sleep are spectacular.

If sleep reduces brain plaques in humans the way it does in mice, then it's a wonder drug indeed. NO drug available from your doctor can do that! Scientists have searched high and low for a drug that reverses brain plaques, and so far they've come up with nothing.

So don't ignore the need for good sleep. Long term chronic sleep-loss changes the brain in ways that make it much more susceptible to brain diseases. Sleep deprivation promotes a vicious cycle where sleep-loss leads to Alzheimer's – and Alzheimer's then leads to even more sleep-loss.

Our health care industry needs to place more emphasis and attention on making sure people get enough quality sleep every night. This is a vital preventative step that works to reduce potential threats to the health of your brain.

Though the typical doctor won't tell you these conditions are linked to brain health, if you suffer from poor digestion… chronic back pain… periodontal disease… and irregular sleep patterns – your brain health is at risk.

RESOURCES AND FURTHER READING:

http://digitaljournal.com/article/319676#ixzz2EcRsVMwP

http://www.livestrong.com/article/140551-brain-exercises-improve-cognition/#ixzz2EO03U1Ys

http://www.losethebackpain.com/blog/2012/05/22/back-pain-may-lead-to-alzheimers/?utm_source=Infusionsoft&utm_medium=Email&utm_content=Alzheimers&utm_campaign=061312_ShortyLeads&inf_contact_key=d928a8531a554c1bff5438ae49db214f04f055123944b89c4b4e8750d6eb758b

http://www.prevention.com/health/brain-games/surprising-tips-boost-your-brain/3-brush-and-floss#ixzz2D462vj3i

http://bebrainfit.com/nutrition/surprising-ways-your-digestive-health-affects-your-brain/

http://www.usnews.com/science/articles/2009/09/24/alzheimers-linked-to-lack-of-sleep

Chapter Two

Is Your Brain Malnourished?

Just as your body needs food to fuel itself and keep you energized throughout the day, your brain requires specific nutrients to ensure it's able to meet all the demands it handles on a daily basis.

A malnourished brain is not something to take lightly. Poor nourishment is rightly considered a brain health hazard.

From the moment of conception all the way up to your golden years, proper nutrients are essential for your brain to operate at its best. Studies even prove malnutrition has a direct bearing on brain function and general health…

In one 2010 study published in the *Social Science & Medicine Journal* a research team, led by Dr. Zhenmei Zhang, studied the data collected from 15,444 elderly Chinese people that were surveyed in regards to their health and longevity.

Researchers found elderly men who suffered from childhood malnourishment had a 29 percent greater risk of experiencing cognitive impairment after age 65 while women in the same age bracket were 35 percent more likely to experience an overall reduction in brain activity.

Your brain is responsible for all the body functions, emotions, and thinking abilities that allow you to live an active and enjoyable life. Failure to provide your brain with the right types of essential vitamins and nutrients can be disastrous for your health and cause permanent – even life changing – damage.

But in order to ensure your brain is getting the right kind of nutritional support, it's important to know what nutrients are "must haves" to experience optimum brain health…

The 3 Basic Things Your Brain *Must* Have

For your brain to reach maximum function, you have to make sure it has a strong foundation. A solid nutrient foundation guarantees that anything else you add or take to further protect your brain can be properly supported and utilized to the full.

Without three vital, basic factors, it is absolutely impossible for the brain to function and survive. So what are these three extremely critical basic needs?

They are water, oxygen and energy. Without them, not even one of the trillions of cells in your body can survive.

Here's how these three basics specifically affect the health of your brain...

Basic Brain Need #1 – Water

Dehydration is a brain killer. This is due to the fact that between 75-80 percent of your brain is water. So keeping your brain well hydrated needs to be a priority if you want to maintain even the most basic level of health.

The effects of dehydration on the brain determine the state of its physical makeup and structure. For example, when brain tissue is deficient in water it begins to shrink. There's even a temporary loss of cognitive function as well.

Studies on dehydration show that if the average person sweats for just 90 minutes without replenishing his or her water supply, the brain will shrink by the equivalent of one year's worth of aging.

This fact has caused a growing number of researchers to believe that Alzheimer's disease is directly linked to the long-term side effects caused by dehydration of the brain. The theory is that by simply maintaining healthy water levels and preventing dehydration the risk for Alzheimer's can be reduced significantly.

Now, most people fall into the typical mindset or practice of only drinking water when they feel thirsty... or when engaging in some form of physical activity... or during meal times. So if these situations aren't present, then the average person rationalizes that they're drinking enough water. Sadly, this mentality helps explain why three out of four Americans today suffer from chronic dehydration, according to some authorities.

The problem is thirst isn't the only way your brain tries to alert you of dehydration. There are more subtle symptoms the brain uses besides thirst that signal a need to re-hydrate. Some of these symptoms include:

• Constipation

• Digestive problems

• High or low blood pressure

• Low energy

Another important point you should know is that your brain requires *water* to stay properly hydrated – not juices... soft drinks... teas... or other beverages. These other liquids cannot match the hydrating power of water. Tea and coffee are diuretics – they actually cause you to excrete water – the opposite of what you need.

Unfortunately, Americans tend to consume large amounts of these other beverages, ignoring the brain's desperate signals that it needs actual water. So if you prefer to drink a variety of other beverages and neglect your water consumption, make it a point to try and include more water when you feel the desire to drink something. Getting back into the habit of regularly drinking water will help you build a stronger foundation for better brain health.

Now for years, doctors and healthcare institutions alike have recommended drinking a minimum of at least 8 glasses of water per day. But there are a variety of factors that require you to drink even more water than that on a daily basis.

The fact is that some days you will exert yourself more than others, which means you'll potentially need more than eight glasses of water. In some cases an active, healthy person may need more than eight glasses – 64 ounces – of water a day to prevent dehydration.

You never want to underestimate your body's need for water – especially when this directly bears on the health of your brain. Make it a point to stay properly hydrated each and every day.

Basic Brain Need #2 – Oxygen

As funny as it may seem, most people use oxygen inefficiently, and as a result the brain suffers.

Medical research shows the brain can only survive for a few minutes without oxygen. Any longer and cells start to die, causing brain activity to cease. In fact, in many trauma situations doctors are constantly checking to make sure the brain is getting an adequate oxygen supply to prevent the patient from becoming brain dead.

Oxygen is a critical component of brain health. Of course, with every breath you take you know your body is getting oxygen. But even though your body is getting oxygen you can still be limiting the amount of oxygen that reaches your brain without even realizing it, thereby preventing it from achieving optimum function.

So how can you improve the flow of oxygen to your brain? Here are five simple breathing tips to help you do just that:

- **Breathe from your diaphragm** – Most people fall into the habit of taking shallow breaths instead of deep breaths. When this occurs, you don't get nearly enough oxygen to improve the brain's capabilities. Shallow breaths limit the amount of oxygen, sometimes to the point where you only get what's absolutely essential to keep you alive. Get into the habit of taking deep breaths that maximize oxygen input, giving your brain a healthy supply to draw from.

- **Check your posture** – Studies show that just by standing up straight lung capacity is increased by five percent. Poor posture can inhibit the flow of oxygen to your brain. By simply correcting the position of your body, you open up a clear path and allow more oxygen to reach your brain.

- **Engage in regular moderate exercise** – Any exercise that increases your heart rate will also increase the flow of oxygen to your brain. Activities like biking… swimming… and walking are great for helping you get your oxygen levels back up where they need to be for normal brain activity. Generally speaking, after moderate exercise people feel good and have more mental clarity. This is partly due to the increased presence of oxygen in the brain. Maintaining a regular exercise program is one of the most important things you can do to keep your brain in good shape and prevent health problems.

- **Limit your exposure to smoke** – People who smoke are at higher risk of having less oxygen flow to their brains. But even if you're exposed to secondhand smoke, there's still a high risk for not getting a sufficient amount of oxygen to your brain. So if you're a smoker – quit! The sooner the better. And if you're exposed to a smoky environment – do what is necessary to limit your exposure, because not doing so will rob your brain of oxygen.

- **Maintain a healthy diet** – A high fat diet actually reduces your blood's oxygen-carrying capacity, which ultimately leads to your brain being starved or deprived of oxygen. However, a diet complete with **complex carbohydrates** will increase your blood's ability to transport oxygen to the brain cells. So make sure your daily diet consists of plenty of fresh fruits and vegetables… whole grains… and legumes to promote a continuous healthy flow of oxygen to the brain. Simple carbohydrates, on the other hand, should be avoided. These include sugar, white flour, white rice and potatoes, which generally raise your blood sugar, add weight in the form of fat, and put you at greater risk of heart disease, diabetes and cancer.

With every breath you take, you want to make sure you're getting the most oxygen that you possible can. Never deprive your brain of this valuable life-saving nutrient!

Basic Brain Need #3 – Energy

Getting plenty of water and oxygen helps create a stable environment for your brain. But the same way a car needs fuel to get you where you need to go, the brain needs energy – and plenty of it – to do its complicated work.

Studies on the function of brain cells **showed these cells in particular need twice the amount of energy of other cells** in order to perform their jobs within the brain properly.

The energy your brain cells feed on comes from sugar – more specifically glucose. But this is NOT a green light to eat lots of table sugar or sugary foods. Keep reading, please!

Your brain requires a constant, steady flow of glucose because brain cells can only survive – at most – several minutes without it. This is because brain cells lack the ability to store glucose in reserve, so they must receive a constant supply readily available to draw from when energy is needed.

Glucose is transported to the brain as blood circulates through the arteries. Now, blood itself does not actually enter into the brain. The arteries create a blood-brain barrier that protects the brain and keeps potential toxins and other substances from entering it. Arteries work like filters by keeping the bad stuff out of the brain and allowing glucose molecules to pass through the artery wall, where they are quickly absorbed and utilized by the brain cells for energy.

Most Americans suffer no shortage of glucose circulating in the blood. Just the opposite: They eat too many carbohydrates. The problem is, they eat the wrong kind. They eat a large amount of simple carbohydrates such as sugar and very few complex carbohydrates such as whole fruit or grains.

Consuming the right foods is important in order for the brain to receive a healthy supply of glucose and avoid blood sugar ups and downs.

Complex carbohydrates such as whole grains, legumes, fresh fruits and vegetables work to stabilize blood sugar levels and also increase the blood's oxygen-carrying capabilities. Thus a proper diet allows the brain to get a constant, steady flow of glucose to the cells that need it most.

It's important to avoid absorbing too much sugar from sweets like candy bars… cookies… or sodas. Although your body does convert them to glucose, the sugar in these foods – either sucrose or fructose – puts the brain at higher risk of becoming energy deficient. These sugary foods provide a short-term energy boost but they do little to help the brain actually maintain stable energy levels.

What's worse, eating these sugary foods on a regular basis triggers high blood sugar levels. Studies show the hippocampus – or the part of the brain that is directly linked to memory function – actually shows *decreased* activity when blood sugar levels are too high.

The three factors we've just covered – water, oxygen, and glucose-based energy – provide the brain with the basics so it can function normally. They can be likened to staple foods needed to keep the brain from starving to death. Being deficient in any one of them can put a crack in the foundation and jeopardize overall brain health and stability.

All the other vitamins, minerals, and nutrients cannot be fully utilized by the brain to perform their specific tasks until these three basic needs have been satisfied.

Four *Must-Have* Nutrients for Your Brain

Studies show that good nutrition throughout your entire life has a direct bearing on brain function. Nutritional neglect or deficiency is often a potential cause of diseases like Alzheimer's and dementia.

If your brain is deficient in certain key nutrients, you run the risk that you will never achieve the peak cognitive abilities you're capable of. Can you imagine not being able to experience certain aspects of life to the full because your brain is missing the one key ingredient that unlocks the door to optimum mental health?

In order to provide your brain with maximum protection from brain diseases… supercharge brain activity… and improve memory and other cognitive functions, there are four vital nutrients you desperately need.

These four unique nutrients are designed to build up your brain's reserve power and keep it fully active at its highest level.

<u>Phosphatidylserine (PS)</u> – This nutrient belongs to the chemical compound group known as phospholipids. All the cells in the body contain trace amounts of PS, but brain cells contain the largest amounts. Because of this, PS is at the top of the list of compounds most beneficial to the brain.

This nutrient is so vital to the brain that numerous double-blind studies have found PS can be an effective treatment to cope with symptoms linked to both Alzheimer's disease and dementia resulting from other causes.

To date, scientists have found PS provides most of its benefits in functions associated with the cellular membrane. The primary responsibilities of PS include keeping brain cell membranes flexible… fluid… and ready to process other essential nutrients.

This amazing nutrient has also been scientifically proven to aid in:

• Cell communication and excitability

• Regulating various neuroendocrine responses

• Releasing acetylcholine, noradrenaline, and dopamine

Further research into the benefits of PS revealed it even influences the response of brain tissue when inflammation is present and can work as a powerful antioxidant to repair damage to the brain caused by such things as free radicals and iron-mediated oxidation.

PS is truly a critical nutrient you need to support healthier brain activity. Unfortunately, symptoms of PS deficiency can start to appear as early in life as the mid 30s.

These are a few symptoms that can indicate insufficient levels of PS:

• Decrease in the ability to learn

• Depression

• Difficulty remembering things

• Struggling to stay and feel mentally alert

In order to combat the effects of PS deficiency it's important to build up your reserves of this nutrient.

Including PS-rich foods – such as fatty fish and organ meats – in your daily diet can help you keep a healthy level of this nutrient in your brain cells.

According to author Parris Kidd, Ph.D, an authority on the nutritional benefits of PS, getting a minimum of at least 300mg of PS a day can help improve brain health… raise PS levels within the brain… and prevent – even reverse – age related decline in brain function.

<u>Alpha-lipoic acid (ALA) and Acetyl L-carnitine (ALC)</u> – These two related nutrients are utilized by the mitochondria in your cells where energy is produced. The mitochondria are responsible for burning food in the presence of oxygen and converting it into energy. They're sometimes called the cell's "energy factories."

Cells that are fully oxidized maintain a much higher level of energy. However, the process of burning and converting food into energy puts the mitochondria at greater risk of free radical damage. In fact, the older you get, the higher the risk that your mitochondria will experience free radical damage.

The damage inflicted by free radicals causes mitochondria to malfunction and severely limits the amount of energy they're able to produce. As you get older, the rate of mitochondrial decay increases, too.

This is disastrous for the brain because, as mentioned earlier, brain cells need twice the amount of energy required by the rest of the body's cells. So malfunctioning mitochondria are a death sentence for brain cells.

That's why it's extra important to make sure you get plenty of ALA and ALC into your body. ALA and ALC in combination work to prevent oxidative damage and also to restore the health, efficiency and integrity of brain cell mitochondria.

The benefits of ALA and ALC on brain rejuvenation are attracting more and more attention from scientists. For example, a recent study conducted on the effects of ALA and ALC on lab rats provided some solid evidence that these two nutrients can help de-age the brain – completely restoring an older person's cognitive faculties to those of a much younger mind…

In this study, a combination of ALA and ALC was administered to old lab rats. The impact these nutrients had on the mice astounded researchers. The old rats began acting like young lab rats. They exhibited the same level of energy and vigor.

Researchers concluded that these two nutrients could potentially provide a person with a fountain of youth that brain cells can draw from in order to sustain the highest level of brain health possible.

Taking ALA and ALC supplements can ultimately help you:

• Improve memory functions relating to space and time

• Reverse problems caused by oxidative stress and cellular aging

• Reduce the number of free radicals present in the brain

• Slow down the deterioration of the mitochondria

It might also be beneficial to add foods containing ALA and ALC to your daily diet. Foods with high amounts of ALA include cruciferous vegetables like broccoli and spinach as well as beef, brewer's yeast and organ meats. ALC is commonly found in meat, dairy products, poultry and fish.

To obtain maximum powerhouse protection from these two nutrients it's best to take them separately, because when combined together in one supplement each is significantly less effective.

Glycerophosphocholine (GPC) – This particular nutrient is a unique phospholipid substance that is of significant importance in improving cognitive function.

Studies on the effects of GPC on brain health reveal that it's an aid in improving:

• Cognitive processing

• Concentration

• Focus

• Memory recall

There have been over 20 clinical trials conducted to gather evidence to support the positive benefits GPC has on the brain. The results, based on more than 4,000 participants, give overwhelming evidence of the multiple benefits of GPC on the brain.

For starters, one double-blind trial reported that adults supplementing with GPC experienced improved reaction time… felt more alert… and were able to focus much better than adults not taking GPC. And according to a review of their brain wave patterns, GPC was the reason for these drastic improvements in overall brain health.

Another trial focused on the restorative benefits of GPC. Using a sample of young people with drug-related memory impairment problems, researchers administered a regular regimen of GPC. Those taking the GPC supplement reported restored memory function and improved concentration capabilities.

When it comes to brain recovery, GPC can help you regain brain functions commonly lost as a result of aging, illness, poor circulation and even injury. This fact has prompted further studies to determine if GPC could be an effective treatment for brain diseases like Alzheimer's and dementia.

During one trial, Alzheimer's patients were administered 1200 mg of GPC for six months. When patients were re-evaluated at the end of that period, they reported significant improvements in behavior, cognition and daily activities.

Five other published trials showed GPC was effective in treating patients recovering from stroke.

In one of these trials, participants who survived a stroke were injected with GPC daily for 30 days and then given an oral GPC supplement for the next five months.

After the initial 30-day period, participants given the injection experienced a 20 to 30 percent recovery of neurological function. During the next five months, participants continued to experience steady improvement in their neurological function.

GPC has proven to be profoundly valuable in achieving maximum brain restoration and better overall health. An intake ranging from 300-1200 mg of GPC in supplement form is an effective way to start restoring healthy levels of GPC in the brain.

As an added benefit to better memory… improved mental clarity… and promoting brain rejuvenation, GPC also works to:

- Improve sociability

- Keep mood levels stable

- Promote a positive attitude

- Revitalize declining mental function

Simply put – the brain needs GPC. You don't want your brain to be deficient in GPC because it's highly effective in optimizing mental focus, memory, and rapid brain repair.

Docosahexaenoic (DHA) – The brain is comprised of 60 percent fat, and 35 to 40 percent of that fat comes from DHA, an omega-3 fatty acid.

Valued as an essential building block to the entire structure of the brain and the retina of the eye, DHA is the most abundant fatty acid naturally produced within the brain. It's actually the only fatty acid that is scientifically linked to reducing the risk of age-related cognitive decline.

DHA's importance in promoting healthy brain activity has made it a center of scientific inquiry…

For starters, it works wonders in improving:

- Brain and nerve function

- Memory

- Mood

- Visual acuity

DHA is a *must-have* nutrient because it naturally works to promote consistent electrical activity from the cellular level up.

All of your brain cells… retinas… and various components inside the nervous system are intricately connected by a network of complex signals that are responsible for transporting electrical messages throughout your entire body. These signals keep the lines of communication open between the brain and the rest of the nervous system.

It's critical that nerve cell membranes get a constant supply of DHA because it is at the membrane level where nerve cells transmit messages and generate electric impulses that are the foundation for all communication that occurs in the nervous system.

A deficiency in DHA causes communication within this intricate system to be broken or interrupted. When this happens, the function of the entire nervous system becomes much less effective than normal.

As you get older, the risk of becoming deficient in DHA is much higher. Aging makes it increasingly difficult for the body to actually make the DHA it needs to enjoy healthy brain function.

Food sources rich in DHA include: High quality eggs… fatty fish such as salmon… red meats… and organ foods.

5 More Essential Nutrients
for Better Memory – and Sharper Thinking

In a recent study it was estimated that roughly 5 million elderly people suffer from some degree of memory malfunction.

Another study found roughly 1 in 6 elderly people over the age of 70 suffer from mild cognitive impairment. Around half of those individuals will end up developing Alzheimer's disease or dementia within 5 years after they receive a diagnosis of mild cognitive impairment.

People suffering from mild cognitive impairment experience problems with memory, language and communication skills, and other mental faculties as well. In the early stages, these symptoms are mild enough not to interfere with daily life, but they become more severe as time goes by.

Specific nutrients are required to keep the memory sharp and thinking abilities active, and to combat the debilitating effects caused by brain diseases associated with aging.

Five nutrients in particular are supported by more than enough evidence to prove they improve memory and thinking power while, at the same time, they lower your risk for brain diseases.

B Vitamins – There are a variety of B vitamins and every last one of them is extremely important in maintaining a good level of health when it comes to your brain and nerves.

One of the noteworthy benefits B vitamins provide is to protect the brain from shrinking and losing volume – one of the common features of old age. Brain shrinking – especially when it becomes severe – is seen in people with Alzheimer's disease and dementia.

B vitamins like folic acid… vitamin B12… and vitamin B6 are known for their ability to control homocysteine levels in the blood. High levels of the amino acid homocysteine are associated with a greater risk of Alzheimer's disease.

During a 2-year randomized clinical trial conducted at Oxford University, researchers focused on the effects of B vitamins in lowering Alzheimer's risk, improving cognitive function, and reducing the rate of age-related brain shrinkage.

In this study, 168 volunteers over age 70 were split into different test groups. One group received a high dose of a B vitamin supplement, while the other received a placebo. Using MRI scans, researchers measured the rate of brain atrophy – or shrinking – over the next two years.

On average, researchers found those taking the B vitamin supplement experienced brain atrophy at a rate of 0.76 percent per year while the placebo group had a 1.08 percent rate of brain atrophy. This translates into a 30 percent reduction in the rate of brain shrinkage every year just by taking B vitamins.

After conducting various memory tests, the researchers found that participants in the study who had the slowest rate of shrinkage scored higher than those in the placebo group. This means the measurable physical symptom – decline in the size of the brain – is directly related to cognitive ability.

The participants with high homocysteine levels were also found to have a much lower atrophy rate after supplementing with B vitamins, compared to those taking the placebo.

Now if the brain atrophy rate is known to be higher in people suffering from mild cognitive impairment, and if B vitamins have proven to slow down the rate at which the brain is getting smaller, then clearly there is a strong possibility B vitamins can help prevent the development and progression of Alzheimer's… dementia… and other brain diseases.

As mentioned before, all the B vitamins are essential for good brain function, but there is one B vitamin that has proven to have tremendous success in a number of studies related to preserving and protecting memory function as well as improving thinking ability…

At Oxford University, a team of scientists studied 107 elderly people ranging from 61 to 81 years old who were not yet suffering from memory problems or impaired thinking abilities. The average age of the participants was 73. Roughly 54 percent of the group were women.

Blood samples of all the participants were collected and studied to check the amount of vitamin B12 present in their bodies. None of the participants were deficient in vitamin B12. The scientists also administered a series of memory tests, an MRI brain scan, and physical examinations.

In comparing the results, researchers found that participants with higher vitamin B12 levels were 6 times less likely to have brain shrinkage compared to those with lower levels of the nutrient in their blood.

In another study – conducted by the Chicago Health and Aging Project – blood samples were taken from 121 seniors over age 65 to measure vitamin B12 levels. The participants were also given various thinking-skill-related tests that measured concentration, short-term memory, and other cognitive processes. MRI brain scans of the participants were taken 4-5 years later.

Scientists studying the data found those who had vitamin B12 deficiency were more likely to have smaller brains and to score lower on the skills tests.

Based on the results from these two studies it is safe to conclude that eating more foods containing B vitamins – especially vitamin B12 – can reduce your risk for brain shrinkage, resulting in better memory function and a lower chance of developing brain diseases.

Sublingual vitamin B12 supplements (i.e. those that dissolve below the tongue) are absorbed and utilized by the body better than those that are swallowed. You can get this high-quality form of B12 on line for as little as four cents a pill.

In one recent Finnish study published in the *Neurology* journal, high doses of B vitamins were used to treat Alzheimer's disease and reduce memory loss symptoms. Researchers found the risk of developing Alzheimer's decreased by 2 percent when levels of B vitamin supplementation were increased.

More recent studies offer solid evidence that supplementing with vitamin B12 can cut the rate of brain shrinkage in elderly people suffering from mild memory and cognitive impairment by 50 percent or more.

Vitamin B12 is a lifesaver for the brain. This nutrient is found primarily in animal foods like eggs… cheese… fortified cereals… meats… and fish. The problem is that after age 50, it starts to become increasingly difficult for the body to naturally absorb vitamin B12 from food sources.

Here's something else important to note about vitamin B12…

Having supposedly normal vitamin B12 levels does not necessarily mean there is enough vitamin B12 in the brain. Associate clinical professor of neurology Dr. Daniel C. Potts, M.D., made the statement that "checking for serum vitamin B12 levels in elderly patients is probably not enough." This is because the presence of vitamin B12 in the blood does not indicate how much is actually in the tissues.

This explains why 15-17 percent of participants in one study whose blood levels measured in the normal range for vitamin B12 still had elevated levels of biomarkers showing they were deficient in this particular nutrient.

Preventing B-vitamin-related deficiencies is critical in improving memory function and maintaining healthy brain volume.

Omega-3 Fatty Acids – The unique properties of omega-3 fatty acids help protect your memory like a force field in a science fiction story. Earlier we mentioned one of the omega-3s, DHA. But numerous studies suggest that a diet rich in a variety of omega-3 fatty acids significantly lowers the risk for Alzheimer's disease and other serious memory problems.

In one study, researchers monitored the diets of 1,219 seniors over age 65 for a year. They then took blood samples from each participant, testing to see if they had the beta-amyloid protein.

High levels of beta-amyloid in the blood have been scientifically linked with mild memory problems as well as full-blown Alzheimer's disease. Studies have found that the plaques and tangles found in the brains of Alzheimer's patients are comprised of the beta-amyloid protein.

Participants in the study who maintained a regular quantity of omega-3 fatty acids in their diets had significantly lower levels of beta-amyloid protein when their blood samples were evaluated.

In fact, researchers found the level of beta-amyloid in participants consuming omega-3s decreased roughly 20-30 percent for each gram of omega-3s added to their diet.

Another study published in the *Medical Journal of the American Academy of Neurology* tested several nutrients – such as vitamin B12, beta-carotene, vitamin D, vitamin E and omega-6 fatty acids – against omega-3s to determine their effects on the beta-amyloid protein.

Out of all the other nutrients studied, omega-3s were the only ones that proved to be effective in lowering beta-amyloid levels.

One further study conducted in 2010 revealed consuming foods high in omega-3 fatty acids lowered the risk for Alzheimer's disease by almost 40 percent.

Some foods rich in omega-3 fatty acids include:

- Fish oil supplements

- Flaxseed (ground, or as fresh flaxseed oil)

- Herring

- Kale

- Mackerel

- Salmon

- Soybeans

- Tofu

- Trout

- Tuna

- Walnuts

According to dietary guidelines, one gram of omega-3 fatty acids can come from about two ounces of salmon or a handful of walnuts. A *minimum* of 2-3 grams of omega-3-rich foods should be consumed on a weekly basis to help guarantee the brain maintains a strong level of these vital nutrients.

<u>Vitamin C</u> – Probably best known for its strong antioxidant capabilities and immune-boosting power, vitamin C is a beneficial nutrient for maintaining a consistent level of good health for your entire body. It's the number one vitamin used to treat and prevent colds, flu, and other sicknesses.

Scientists and medical professionals have all seen and understood the importance of vitamin C in making sure a person has healthy bones, teeth, cartilage, and tissues. However, more and more research is being published that provides solid evidence the brain utilizes vitamin C for a variety of other purposes as well.

For starters, vitamin C acts as an enzyme helper – aiding in the synthesis of the brain neurotransmitters: epinephrine, dopamine, and norepinephrine. These neurotransmitters are responsible for carrying instructions to the other parts of the body to perform their respective tasks.

Vitamin C regulates these neurotransmitters, preventing them from speeding up cellular communication and overworking brain cells. An imbalance in this area can cause serious brain cell damage to the point where the cells actually work themselves to death. Without adequate amounts of vitamin C, the entire chemistry of the brain can be altered, resulting in a variety of brain-related health problems.

Another benefit to vitamin C is that it plays a critical role in the formation of collagen – the main component of connective tissues in the body. Collagen is also the substance that surrounds the myelin sheath – or lining – around your sensitive and delicate nerves.

Healthy collagen is vital in keeping the structure of the brain strong. Fortifying collagen with an increase of vitamin C can help prevent brain hemorrhages – especially among the elderly.

Vitamin C fights dangerous free radicals that constantly try to attack brain cells and weaken overall brain health. If sufficient vitamin C is made available to the brain, the potential risk of damage posed by free radicals is significantly reduced

The brain cannot sustain strong structural integrity without vitamin C. But this nutrient is also vital in combating memory-loss symptoms typical of Alzheimer's disease.

Studies conducted on Alzheimer's patients showed the majority have very low levels of vitamin C. Many had outright vitamin C deficiency.

In clinical trials conducted on mice, scientists found that those suffering from memory loss – associated with both Alzheimer's disease and dementia in humans – had a reversal of their symptoms when administered a regular dose of vitamin C daily.

Yet, sadly, the Centers for Disease Control recently reported that one man out of ten is vitamin C deficient.

Vitamin C deficiency severely affects overall brain health. Brain studies reveal the amount of vitamin C in the brain is roughly four times higher than the level of vitamin C in the bloodstream. Clearly, the brain has a high need for this vitamin. That's why it reacts strongly when it lacks this nutrient.

If a person suffers from vitamin C deficiency, the brain does everything it can to protect its own supply of vitamin C from being used or absorbed by other parts of the body.

Vitamin C is one of the few vitamins your body does not naturally produce on its own. So you need to ensure that you get a regular supply of vitamin C by either supplementation or diet.

According to various governmental health agencies, for the average person, a recommendation of 90 mg as a daily minimum amount of vitamin C is sufficient for good health. Most nutritionists regard that level as pitifully low, and recommend an intake of at least 500 to 1000 mg per day.

To guarantee your brain will never have to go without this vital nutrient, it's advisable to supplement with a higher dosage. There's no toxicity associated with high levels of vitamin C.

Some people report diarrhea at extremely high doses – for example, 10,000 milligrams per day – but the diarrhea stops when the dose is reduced to a more reasonable level. Some people report stomach upset at fairly low doses, and there are buffered forms of vitamin C to help prevent this side effect. You should have no problem at 1000 mg per day of a buffered product, and most people can tolerate two or three times that much with no stomach upset.

An adequate amount is also easy to get through diet by including a variety of foods naturally rich in vitamin C. Foods containing high amounts of vitamin C include:

- Broccoli

- Cantaloupe

- Dark leafy green vegetables

- Kiwi

- Oranges and other citrus fruit

- Strawberries

- Watermelon

Always remember to monitor your intake of vitamin C so you never have to worry that your brain is missing out on its protective benefits.

Vitamin D – From the very early stages of life, vitamin D plays a role in the development of the human brain. Studies of the beginning stages of pregnancy reveal high concentrations of vitamin D are present, especially at critical stages of brain development.

Within the brain are vitamin D receptors and enzymes that are responsible for converting the 25-hydroxy form of vitamin D, also known as calcidiol, into calcitriol. The calcitriol form of vitamin D is then responsible for altering the expression of numerous genes within brain cells. This directly affects certain proteins inside the brain responsible for helping nerve cells survive and become specialized to their individual jobs.

Vitamin D has to be a constant presence in order for the brain to develop properly. A deficiency in this nutrient can severely alter and limit how well the brain functions.

Vitamin D deficiency is determined by measuring how much of this nutrient is present in the bloodstream. This blood test is known as the 25-hydroxy vitamin D blood test. 25 to 50 ng/mL (nanograms/milliliter) is considered a healthy amount of vitamin D. A level less than 12 ng/mL is a strong indication of vitamin D deficiency.

Low blood levels of vitamin D can increase the risk for cognitive decline, dementia, and other brain-related problems.

The *Archives of Internal Medicine* reported the findings of a 6-year study where researchers collected data from 858 seniors aged 65 and older to determine the effects of vitamin D on cognitive function.

Participants were required to complete the standard test known as the Mini-Mental State Examination or MMSE as well as two other tests to properly assess their cognitive performance in relation to attention, planning, organizing, and overall cognitive skill.

The tests revealed that, in comparison to the group of participants with normal vitamin D levels, those who had vitamin D levels less than 25 nmol/L – indicating a clear deficiency – had an alarming 60 percent greater risk for substantial cognitive decline as measured by the MMSE. According to the other assessment tests, the vitamin-D-deficient participants had a 30 percent greater risk of cognitive decline.

Based on this study, researchers concluded low levels of vitamin D were strongly associated with substantial cognitive decline among the elderly.

In regards to brain diseases like dementia and Alzheimer's, scientific evidence is now pointing to the possible role vitamin D plays in the early onset of Alzheimer's disease. In fact, Alzheimer's patients have low levels of vitamin D in comparison to healthy people.

Further studies showed Alzheimer's patients with poor vitamin D levels had much lower scores on their cognitive tests than those with adequate D levels. Researchers believe the anti-inflammatory and immune-boosting properties of vitamin D can combat the inflammation-triggered symptoms of Alzheimer's disease.

And even more noteworthy were the positive results seen when patients suffering from Alzheimer's were given vitamin D as a daily supplement. Their performance on tests of cognitive ability improved.

Diet and supplementation are the most effective ways to increase the amount of vitamin D in the blood and prevent deficiency.

Guidelines published by the Institute of Medicine recommended a dietary allowance of 600 international units (IU) of vitamin D for people aged 61-70 years and 800 IU daily for seniors over 80 years of age. Those dosages are minimal. Older people can and should take 2000 IU per day.

A recent list of vitamin D guidelines published by the *Canadian Medical Association Journal* suggested that those under age 50 should get between 400-1000 IU of vitamin D and those over age 50 should aim to have a daily intake of 800-2000 IU of vitamin D.

These are just basic guidelines. Ten years ago, the medical establishment was saying – wrongly – that 400 IU per day was the maximum safe dose. A blood test is the proper way to determine how much vitamin D you require. A blood test will help you determine whether or not you need to increase your daily intake of vitamin D until your blood levels of this nutrient reach the desired level of 25 to 50 ng/mL. Reaching that level may require months of taking high-dose vitamin D supplements, if your current blood level is extremely low.

Foods that contain vitamin D include:

- Beef liver

- Cheese

- Egg yolks

- Fish

- Fish oils

- Fortified milk (with D added)

- Milk

You can also increase your body's natural production of vitamin D by spending more time in the sun. It's rightly nicknamed "the sunshine vitamin."

Allowing your skin to absorb healthy rays from the sun is the cheapest way to increase vitamin D levels – yet it is often the most challenging due to different skin types… climate… and geographical locations.

A word of caution: If you are going to spend more time in the sun, be sure to take good care of your skin so you avoid sunburn and skin damage. As little as 10 or 15 minutes of sun per day during the summer is enough to help your body produce a very large amount of vitamin D.

During other seasons, more time in the sun is required, and the farther north you live, the less intense the sunlight, especially in fall, winter and spring. All these factors influence the amount of time you can spend in the sun without skin damage.

<u>Vitamin E</u> – This nutrient is stored in the fat of the body. It is made up of a group of fat-soluble compounds that are known to have strong antioxidant properties. Foods like wheat germ… vegetable oils… leafy green vegetables… whole grains… nuts… and seeds all contain ample amounts of vitamin E.

Vitamin E is like a strong shield for the brain because it protects brain cells from free radical damage that can ultimately contribute to the development of brain diseases. The brain naturally has a high rate of oxygen consumption and a high amount of polyunsaturated fatty acids within its neuronal cell membranes.

Over time, free radicals can cause serious damage to the brain's neurons, increasing the risk for cognitive decline, memory problems, and neurodegenerative diseases like Alzheimer's.

The antioxidant properties of vitamin E work to stop these free radicals before they have a chance to cause long-term damage to the brain.

In one study conducted over a 3-year period, consuming vitamin E contributed in a large way to a decrease in cognitive decline in participants aged 65-102.

But there are other benefits that can be derived from vitamin E as well...

In 2004, *The New England Journal of Medicine* published a study reviewing natural therapies – including antioxidants – to treat Alzheimer's disease. The review included studies in which vitamin E along with selegiline – a drug used to treat symptoms linked to Parkinson's – was administered to people suffering from Alzheimer's and dementia.

In one double-blind, randomized study, 341 patients suffering from Alzheimer's disease were administered 2000 IU of vitamin E to determine its benefits (if any) to cognitive function.

During this 2-year study, participants were split into several test groups and received one of the following:

- 2000 IU of vitamin E daily

- A placebo

- Both vitamin E and selegiline

- Selegiline – A monoamine oxidase inhibitor medication commonly used to treat Parkinson's disease.

The study revealed that those treated with vitamin E or selegiline or both at the same time delayed the deterioration usually associated with the progression of Alzheimer's disease. A decline in day-to-day performance of routine activities and the increase in the amount of care needed were both significantly delayed for participants in those test groups.

Another clinical trial found similar benefits to vitamin E in the treatment of brain diseases. During this trial, patients classified with moderate Alzheimer's disease had a slower rate of functional decline, a finding similar to that in the study described above.

Scientists believe with these kinds of positive benefits vitamin E could help prevent dementia in elderly people who are in the early stages of the disease and have not yet experienced severe cognitive impairment.

Encouraged by these studies, some doctors are now choosing to add 2000 IU of vitamin E to their standard treatment plan for Alzheimer's disease and dimentia.

Your Brain Desperately Needs All These Nutrients

More and more research is showing that a combination of all the essential nutrients mentioned above is vital in sustaining increased brain function and improving cognitive activity.

For example, a team of researchers from the Center for Cellular Neurobiology and Neurodegenerative Research used a combination of nutrient additives to determine how much neuroprotection they provide.

The nutrients used in this study were: *Alpha-lipoic acid, acetyl L-carnitine, glycophosphocholine, DHA (an omega-3 fatty acid found in fish oil and other foods)* and *phosphatidylserine (usually called PS).*

These 5 nutrients were regularly administered to mice that were eating a vitamin-free, oxidative-challenged and iron-enriched diet.

Researchers discovered using this supplement reduced reactive oxygen species by 57 percent and also prevented the increase of reactive oxygen species. Supplementing with these nutrients actually prevented the cognitive decline that was found in the control group of mice in this study that were not fed the five-nutrient combo.

This study also adds weight to the importance of adequate brain nutrition and highlights how key nutrients are needed to improve overall performance and prevent brain damage. Without the constant protection of these nutrients, a variety of destructive forces have an opening to inflict damage on brain health.

Another study examined the short-term memory improvements linked to regular supplementation with *phosphatidylserine (PS), vitamin B6, ginkgo biloba,* and *vitamin E.*

Researchers from the University of Toronto conducted a study to determine if commercially available dietary supplements designed to protect neuron tissue could be shown to improve cognitive function.

A group of aged beagles were split into two groups. The first group was the control group and the second group received supplements of PS, vitamin B6, ginkgo biloba and vitamin E.

The researchers quickly discovered that performance on neuropsychological tests of both visual-spatial and short-term memory drastically improved in the aged dogs taking the nutrient supplements. Even better, the benefits were long-lasting – adding weight to the theory that regular supplementation provides long-term brain health benefits.

The Oregon Brain Aging Study provides further evidence to prove the importance of giving the brain a constant supply of all these essential nutrients.

In this study, 104 elderly people – averaging age 87 – with a low risk for both Alzheimer's disease and dementia were examined. At the initial diagnosis, participants were found to have a good level of overall nutrition. However, 7 percent were classified as having low levels of B vitamins and vitamin D.

The participants who maintained adequate levels of omega-3… vitamins C, D, and E… and B vitamins, scored better on thinking tests and also had a lower risk of brain atrophy than did those deficient in these nutrients.

Making it a point to provide your brain with the right nutritional support is more than half the battle in preventing age-related cognitive decline and debilitating brain diseases. Without good nutrition, you risk starving your brain into poor health. The wisest course appears to be to take all the supplements recommended in this chapter rather than pick and choose among them.

Each one has been demonstrated to improve overall brain health and enhance a variety of cognitive functions. Lacking even one of these nutrients may limit your ability to experience optimum brain health. All the supplements recommended in this chapter are easily found at retail stores that sell supplements and on the Internet.

The next chapter will discuss some unique whole *foods* that have been proven beneficial in supplying solid nutrient support to the brain…

RESOURCES AND FURTHER READING:

http://www.livestrong.com/article/479663-how-malnutrition-affects-the-brain/

http://www.wisegeek.org/what-are-free-radicals.htm

http://www.naturalnews.com/025616_brain_nutrients_supplement.html#ixzz2D46dsoFa

http://www.alzinfo.org/04/articles/prevention-and-wellness/5-nutrients-promote-brain-health

http://thechart.blogs.cnn.com/2012/05/02/omega-3-may-curb-memory-loss-study-says/

http://www.forbes.com/sites/daviddisalvo/2012/10/29/new-study-shows-that-omega-3-supplements-can-boost-memory-in-young-adults/

http://www.umm.edu/altmed/articles/omega-3-000316.htm#ixzz2DY0VIv9N

http://www.webmd.com/brain/news/20080908/vitamin-b12-boasts-brain-benefits

http://www.aarp.org/health/brain-health/info-10-2011/b12-level-affects-brain-size-health-discovery.html

http://www.sciencedaily.com/releases/2010/09/100912213050.htm

http://www.newsmaxhealth.com/dr_blaylock/vitamin_C_brain/2012/03/22/440910.html

http://news.menshealth.com/the-vitamin-that-protects-your-brain/2011/07/20/

http://www.webmd.com/diet/vitamin-d-deficiency?page=2

http://www.dummies.com/how-to/content/examining-vitamin-ds-effect-on-the-brain.html

http://jonnybowdenblog.com/can-vitamin-d-protect-your-brain/

http://www.crnusa.org/vitaminEandbrainfunction.html

http://ods.od.nih.gov/factsheets/VitaminE-HealthProfessional/

Chapter Three

Five Superfoods Specially Selected for Your Brain

Can the foods you eat really help you achieve a high level of protection for your brain? Can merely eating right give your brain the strength to fight off diseases and other negative influences that cause your memory and thinking ability to gradually fade away?

According to a study in *Neurology*, a journal published by the American Academy of Neurology, people with high levels of trans fats – mostly from eating a diet of processed, fried or frozen foods, packaged baked goods, and fast foods – scored much lower on memory and thinking tests than people with low levels of trans fats.

The foods that make up your diet play a direct role in how well the brain will function over time. But how can you know for sure whether the foods you eat are helping or harming brain health?

It's easy to tell a doctor or nutritionist what you eat, but this doesn't show for certain how many nutrients are being absorbed into your body. Taking blood measurements of specific nutrients, however, can accurately assess which nutrients may be missing in order to help you add the right foods to your diet and fix any nutrient deficiencies.

Numerous studies point to the positive benefits linked to diets rich in fresh fruits and vegetables… whole grains… and healthy protein-based foods. A well-balanced diet is critical for keeping the brain nourished.

In fact, studies on the health benefits related to specific foods suggest that making simple diet changes can help prevent brain atrophy and give you the gift of a sharper and more active mind.

To help give your brain a strong boost of nutrient power, here are five unique brain superfoods known to improve… enhance… repair… restore… and revitalize the health of the brain:

Brain Superfood #1 – Turmeric

Using turmeric to spice up your meals gives them a burst of flavor. But it's also a unique way to improve the health of the brain. In fact, **simply adding a small amount of curry to just one meal once a month delivers a potent dose of antioxidants directly to the brain.**

First and foremost, the antioxidants found in turmeric (a common ingredient in curry powder) fight against free radicals and the damage they inflict on the brain's cells.

The most powerful antioxidant identified in turmeric is called curcumin, available as a food supplement if you don't eat spicy, turmeric-flavored dishes. This antioxidant works to combat the dangerous effects of inflammation, which is also caused by free radicals.

Studies have found curcumin inhibits the production of COX-2 – a known trigger for inflammation – blocking it from attacking soft tissue all over the body including the brain. In fact, curcumin works just as well – if not better – than pain medications prescribed to manage severe inflammation symptoms. The difference is that with curcumin there is no risk of dangerous side effects.

So by adding some curry powder or pure turmeric to your meals, you can slow down the damaging effects of brain aging and keep normal cognitive function as you enter into your later years.

Brain Superfood #2 – Oysters

Oysters can be a strong memory booster and improve many of the brain's important cognitive functions.

The secret ingredient in oysters that makes them a true brain-boosting superfood is the mineral zinc.

Numerous studies have proven zinc has tremendous benefits in:

• Improving skin tone

• Fighting cancer

• Reducing the length of time a cold lasts

• Speeding up wound healing

But now there is irrefutable evidence showing the high concentration of zinc in oysters can be just what the doctor ordered when it comes to supporting cognitive stability and memory function.

High concentrations of zinc are deposited in those parts of nerve cells called vesicles. The vesicles package neurotransmitters that give nerve cells their ability to communicate. Neurons in the hippocampus (a part of the brain) contain the highest concentration of zinc. These brain neurons are responsible for controlling functions related to learning and memory.

Animal studies conducted by researchers at Duke University Medical Center and chemists from the Massachusetts Institute of Technology revealed some noteworthy benefits zinc has on the brain…

Experimenting with mice, scientists used a chemical that binds with zinc to eliminate it from their brains. Once the animals' brains were depleted of zinc, scientists noticed immediate changes to brain activity.

Communication between brain neurons diminished significantly. The researchers also noted that without zinc, nerve cell function no longer operated as efficiently as it had when zinc was present in the brain. Researchers then concluded that zinc is a key nutrient that plays an intricate role in overall brain communication as well as in cellular and nerve function.

A later stage of the study showed that once zinc levels were increased back to normal, brain communication within the affected hippocamal region of the brain improved; both memory and learning capabilities improved dramatically.

Zinc deficiency is a proven cause for:

• Cognitive decline

• Decline in sexual health

• Difficulty with concentration

• Higher risk for dementia

• Lack of focus

• Memory lapses

• Poor immune function

A proper intake of zinc is a vital step toward achieving optimal brain function and preventing cognitive decline linked to aging.

As mentioned, oysters are extremely rich in zinc. In fact, they are the richest food source for zinc. Depending on the type and variety, oysters can provide anywhere from 16-182mg of zinc per 100g serving.

Steamed Wild Eastern Oysters provide a higher amount of zinc than any other type of oyster studied. As a practical matter, most of us aren't going to eat oysters every day or even every week, so a zinc supplement is appropriate.

Brain Superfood #3 – Dark Chocolate

Chocolate can be your best friend – or your worst enemy. Chocolate can be a so-called "guilty pleasure"… or a sweet treat once in a while… or the main reason you have to battle to keep your weight down. But in spite of the negative aura that surrounds chocolate – dark chocolate actually offers strong support to the brain.

Milk chocolate is popular because it's sweet, but it lacks the nutritious brain nutrients that are abundant in dark chocolate. Though both milk chocolate and dark chocolate contain cocoa and cocoa derivatives, milk chocolate's other ingredients, including sugar and milk, strip away the potential brain-boosting benefits. Dark chocolate may contain sugar as well. Unsweetened or bitter dark chocolate is healthier.

A study from the University of California found you can reap some valuable benefits by consuming dark chocolate.

For starters, dark chocolate helps guard against lipid (fat) peroxidation, which is responsible for altering and destroying the fat membranes of brain cells and can trigger blood fats to become toxic.

Further evidence showed people who eat dark chocolate have a longer life expectancy and a better sense of overall wellbeing.

The core ingredient in chocolate is cocoa. Surprisingly, cocoa is very nutritious for the brain. Scientific studies indicate that 2-3 tablespoons of cocoa powder contain more potent antioxidant capabilities than do other well known antioxidant-rich foods.

The cocoa used to produce dark chocolate is packed full of powerful flavanols – a group of natural compounds that support healthy circulation.

Over 140 scientific studies have been conducted on cocoa flavanols. They show that consumption of these flavanols can help generate improved cognitive function.

In one double blind, controlled study, conducted by Dr. Giovambattista Desideri and a team of researchers from the University of L'Aquila in Italy, regular consumption of cocoa flavanols had positive effects on cognitive function in senior adults suffering from mild cognitive impairment or MCI. MCI is sometimes called "early stage" dementia or Alzheimer's disease.

A person suffering from MCI experiences memory loss to a much greater extent than does a healthy person in the same age group. However, MCI does not usually interfere with everyday activities. Roughly 20 percent of adults over age 65 have MCI.

Studies show that, in recent years, six percent of adults between the ages of 70 and 89 develop MCI each year.

During the study led by Dr. Desideri, 90 older adults diagnosed with MCI were randomly assigned to drink a cocoa flavanol product daily that contained either:

- **HF Group:** High amounts of cocoa flavanols (990 mg)

- **IF Group:** Intermediate amounts of cocoa flavanols (520 mg)

- **LF Group:** Low amounts of cocoa flavanols (45 mg)

No other changes were made to the participants' daily diet that would affect this study.

After 8 weeks, the research team administered a series of tests to examine memory, global cognition, cognitive processing speed, and executive (decision-making) function.

Those who received high or intermediate amounts of cocoa flavanols displayed significant improvement…

Their results showed a 30 percent reduction in response time based on tests that focused on working memory, processing speed and executive function. On the Verbal Fluency Tests (VFT) scores were much higher as well.

Within the low flavanol group there was no evidence of improvement or noticeable difference in performance at the end of the study, compared to the beginning.

Researchers also noted both the high and intermediate groups experienced a reduction in insulin resistance and improvement in glucose metabolism. They felt this benefit played an influential role in the positive effects seen in cognitive function.

The results of this study point to the possibility that consuming dark chocolate can slow down – even reverse – the effects linked to age-related cognitive decline and provide other long-term health benefits as well.

The results support the theory that daily consumption of cocoa flavanols – especially among older adults – can offer valuable benefits to brain health.

Brain Superfood #4 – Tea

For centuries, tea has been a staple part of the diet in many ancient cultures. From early on, regular tea drinking has always been associated with achieving better health and a longer life.

Now, more in-depth studies and research have revealed that freshly brewed green or black tea can be a true secret weapon to help keep the memory fresh, sharp, active and functioning properly.

Tea enriches the brain with catechins – potent phytochemicals and antioxidants that promote good health. This tea ingredient identified by modern science is thought to be the reason tea is a brain superfood.

Catechins from green tea have 100 times the antioxidant power of vitamin C – and 25 times the potency of vitamin E.

Medical research dating back to the 1990s has proven catechins are valuable in promoting better health in a variety ways. For example, laboratory tests reveal catechins found in tea leaves prevent and stop the growth of cancer cells. They also work to combat the dangerous effects linked to free radical damage. Inhibiting free radical activity can significantly lower your risk of cancer and other serious brain diseases.

A review of studies published in a 2006 issue of *Life Sciences* reported evidence that catechins are effective in:

- Preventing tumor blood vessel growth

- Inhibiting the build-up of artery plaque

- Lowering Alzheimer's and Parkinson's disease risk

- Promoting insulin resistance

Smaller amounts of catechins are found in apples… dark chocolate… berries… and even red wine. But tea offers perhaps the best and most potent amounts of these nutrients. Unfermented green tea consists of 27 percent catechins… while semi-fermented Oolong tea contains 23 percent… and black tea has just 4 percent. Green tea has considerably greater nutritional value than black tea. Black tea is fermented tea – the two terms mean the same thing.

When you're feeling tired or mentally drained, low levels of catechins in the brain could be the cause. Catechins are essential for fighting mental fatigue, keeping the memory sharp, and helping the brain learn when to naturally relax so you don't become as tired and rundown.

Drinking a cup of green tea in the morning can help give the brain a healthy boost to perform better in a number of ways.

Brain Superfood #5 – Eggs

According to a study published in the *American Journal of Clinical Nutrition*, the nutrient **choline** – naturally found in eggs – can reduce the risk of dementia.

In this study, 1,400 adults were examined and administered a series of memory tests. Researchers found participants with the highest levels of choline in their blood scored much higher on the tests and had a much lower risk of blood vessel disease. This is noteworthy because blood vessel disease is a major contributing factor for dementia.

Choline is responsible for creating **acetylcholine** – an important neurotransmitter vital to memory activity and other mental functions. It's essential to the function of brain cells and indeed the whole nervous system.

Dietary studies show 5 boiled eggs contain 550 mg of choline – the daily amount the average man needs to maintain good brain health. The yolk has the highest concentration of choline. Eating just one or two eggs a day contributes significantly to brain health.

Eggs can also help fight against brain atrophy, thanks to two other nutrients they contain:

vitamin B12 and lecithin. Thus, eggs also work to lower your risk for Alzheimer's, as brain atrophy increases the risk for this disease.

Including these five superfoods in your diet will help ensure you enjoy maximum brain power as you age.

RESOURCES AND FURTHER READING:

http://www.toptenz.net/top-10-foods-for-brain-health.php#ixzz2D442Dm3K

http://www.shape.com/healthy-eating/diet-tips/11-best-foods-your-brain

http://www.healthaliciousness.com/articles/zinc.php#ge5iQHXvF8HHgOUy.99

http://www.naturalnews.com/033722_zinc_memory.html#ixzz2DkZfAFzT

http://www.terrysmall.com/bb_40.asp

http://www.alzheimersreadingroom.com/2012/08/cocoa-flavanol-consumption-shown-to.html

http://www.livestrong.com/article/478075-foods-high-in-catechins/#ixzz2Dpn2UsKY

http://www.wisegeek.com/what-are-catechins.htm

Chapter Four

Exercise Your Body –
And Boost Your Mind, Too!

A regular exercise routine will not only keep you in shape and feeling good, but can also promote healthier brain activity – and make you smarter too!

According to associate professor of psychiatry and author of *A User's Guide to the Brain*, John J. Ratey, MD, "Exercise is really for the brain, not the body. It affects mood, vitality, alertness and feelings of well-being."

Dozens of studies reviewed by researchers from Beckman Institute found aerobic exercise was very effective in boosting overall mental sharpness and the speed at which the brain processes thoughts. It also helps increase brain tissue volume – a key factor in preventing dementia and Alzheimer's.

These specific benefits were seen in participants who spent a minimum of 50 minutes, three times a week engaging in moderate walking exercise.

Another study showed that walking in parks or some other tree-filled environment helped participants score 20 percent higher on memory and attention tests compared to participants who walked in city areas.

A University of San Francisco fitness and wellness coordinator, Christin Anderson, explained how exercise works to train the brain: Exercise plays a direct role in many of the sites in the nervous system. Neurotransmitters (brain chemicals) like dopamine and serotonin – which are responsible for allowing you to experience happiness, a sense of calm, and feelings of euphoria – are directly affected by the amount of exercise you do on a regular basis.

Exercise can even help reactivate brain activity that has slowed down as a result of aging…

Recently scientists in Brazil have studied the effects exercise had on elderly rats with sedentary patterns of behavior. Scientists had these rats run for roughly 5 minutes, several days a week for the duration of five weeks.

The data received from the test subjects showed biochemical processes within the memory region of the brain surged to higher levels after each session of exercise. Overall production in brain-derived neurotrophic factor (BDNF) molecules also significantly increased. BDNF is a key factor in promoting better nerve cell health and improving memory and skill task performance capabilities.

When these results were compared to the memory tests of the younger rats, the data showed the elderly rats performed almost as well.

A similar animal study performed by researchers from the Brain Injury Research Center at the University of California found adult rats that ran at will for a week had more BDNF molecules in their memory faculties than sedentary rats. And these adult rats also had a higher concentration of precursor molecules that will quickly develop into healthy, fully functioning BDNF molecules.

Based on these studies, regular exercise is a requirement for good brain health. Low or moderate exercise – frequent walks, for example – is adequate.

Depending on your personal lifestyle, aim for 8-12 minutes of daily exercise that increases your heart rate and causes you to sweat. Or you might find it beneficial to engage in 30 minutes of moderate exercise three or more times a week. Hiking, swimming, and walking are all proven forms of exercise that promote better brain and cognitive activity.

New preliminary animal studies even point to regular exercise as a cause for the growth of new, healthy stem cells that can ultimately refresh the brain back into a more youthful state. Exercise also works to stimulate various nerve growth factors as well.

This finding is so important, you need to know more about it. . .

You Can Actually Grow New Brain Cells

For years we've been told that brain loss was an inevitable part of aging… that we automatically lose neurotransmitters as we move on through life.

Until now the medical community has denied the possibility that adult brain cells could regrow.

Now researchers know that neurogenesis – the process of brain cell regeneration or regrowth – *does* occur. And it plays a pivotal role in releasing stress, preventing Alzheimer's, dementia, and depression, and keeping your body's brain and nervous system – your "master control" system – in tip-top shape.

Best of all, you can enjoy all these wonderful benefits for free – with no damaging side effects, because it turns out that **exercise** – not medications and not even foods or supplements – may be the best single way to regrow your brain cells.

Exercise is the secret that can be the difference between aging in your own home, versus moving to an assisted living facility.

Once you've heard the exciting new findings about growing new brain tissue, I'm sure you'll be more than ready to make the effort. You'll want to see these results in your own life, whatever it takes.

By the way, the effort required to regrow your brain isn't all that much. You don't have to be an exercise fanatic. And a small bit of moderate exercise will not only boost your brain, but reduce your risk of heart disease and cancer while you're at it.

So, jog your brain a bit...

Experts now say your brain is no different than your muscles. You either use it or lose it. It's now well established that exercise bolsters both the structure and function of your brain.

Not only is exercise a smart thing to do for your heart and weight – it can literally make you smarter.

It increases your heart rate, oxygenating your brain. Scientists think this oxygen flow helps reduce your brain's free radicals. One of the exciting findings of recent decades is that these inflows are almost always accompanied by an uptick in mental sharpness.

Exercising also fuels "plasticity" to encourage growth of new connections between cells in your brain's cortical areas. Plasticity or neuroplasticity is the scientific term for the brain's ability to change and grow throughout your life – in contrast to the outdated view that the brain is a static, unchanging organ.

Recent research from UCLA shows that exercise increases growth factors in your brain – inducing the growth of new neuron connections.

Best growth stimulant for your brain

Stephen C. Putnam, MEd, embraced canoeing in a serious way to combat adult ADHD. He followed it up by writing a book called *Nature's Ritalin for the Marathon Mind*, in which he writes about the benefits of exercise on hyperactivity and the inability to focus on tasks.

Putnam cites studies of children who ran around for fifteen to 45 minutes before class and thereby cut their squirminess in half *during* class. Their running benefits lasted for two to four hours after exercising.

Putnam also cites preliminary animal research suggesting that exercise may cause new stem cells to grow – enabling your brain to refresh itself. Putnam calls it "Miracle-Gro" for the brain. And it appears there's plenty of science to confirm his observations.

Is exercise the easiest way on earth to reduce stress?

Have you ever heard of "runner's high"?

Scientists know that exercise releases a rush of hormones that discharge pleasure chemicals – including two that were mentioned earlier, serotonin and dopamine. Both these natural neurotransmitters make you feel calm, happy, or euphoric…

In other words, runner's high is like an all-natural antidepressant. Prescription medications for depression actually aim to increase the body's level of serotonin, but you don't need the drugs, because exercise can accomplish the same feat. Plus "runner's high" does something else: It's linked to a drop in stress hormones.

A study out of Stockholm showed that **"runner's high" also stimulates new cell growth in the hippocampus – the part of your brain responsible for learning and memory**.

So if you don't want to wait around for good feelings to happen on their own. . .and if you don't want to induce them with a prescription drug. . .you can nearly always bring them on by exercising.

This is valuable information, because stress does enormous damage to your brain, as you'll see in Chapter Seven.

"First aid" for your brain

Researchers are finding that those who exercise later in life help protect their brain from age-related degeneration more than those who don't exercise. But it gets even better. Exercise may also act like a soothing balm for aging or damaged brain cells.

In a large brain-imaging study done at the University of Edinburgh in Scotland, researchers found a strong and direct correlation over a 3-year period showing that **as physical activity increased, brain shrinkage decreased.**

This study tapped into a highly respected longitudinal aging study, the Lothian Birth Cohort Study. It looked at 638 adults between 70 and 73 years old.

How to Keep Iron Levels in Check

Here are four ways to prevent excessive iron accumulation in your blood:

• **Avoid eating iron-fortified foods** – Foods claiming to be fortified with iron are actually much more dangerous than foods naturally high in iron. Fortified iron is inorganic, meaning your body will have a more difficult time digesting it and sending it where you need it most. As a result, your blood will contain higher amounts of iron. Processed foods like white breads and cereals are some of the most widely-consumed foods that are likely to be fortified with iron. Learn to read ingredient labels to check if a food is iron-fortified.

• **Don't over-supplement** – If you take a variety of vitamin and mineral supplements you might be getting much more iron than you think. Both types of supplements often contain iron. Again, read the list of ingredients. Taking such a supplement may raise your iron to toxic levels. You don't need an iron supplement unless a doctor has given you a blood test and found you're deficient in this mineral. Women are more likely to be iron-deficient than men. A man who consumes red meat regularly almost certainly does not need more iron.

• **Limit the use of iron pots and pans** – Cooking foods – especially acidic foods – in iron pots and pans causes higher amounts of iron to be consumed through your diet. Acidic foods absorb iron from the pot or pan thereby increasing iron levels.

• **Watch your drinking water** – Well water often has high amounts of iron naturally present. So if you drink well water, be sure the house or building's water system has some type of iron precipitator or a reverse osmosis water filter to reduce iron levels.

They found that those who walked several times a week had less brain shrinkage, and fewer signs of brain aging in general, than did the less active folks.

On the other hand, this study found **no** benefit on brain size for participating in socially or mentally stimulating activities. So if you want to maximize the mind-enriching benefits of playing chess or piano, walk or run across town to do it.

This study indicates that exercise is an important "medicine" to keep your brain's size healthy and reduce brain damage as you age.

The brain scans showed that those who were more active had less damage to their white matter (the wiring that sends messages around your brain) and had more grey matter (the part containing nerve cell bodies).

Study participants provided details of their daily activities, ranging from basic chores to engaging in heavy exercise or competitive sports – as well as non-physical leisure activities.

Those most devoted to exercise showed better brain circuitry connections and less brain shrinkage – regardless of initial IQ or social class.

Dementia plummets by almost three-fourths

A group of American researchers looked at the part of the brain called the hippocampus, your brain's memory center.

They followed adults over 65 years old… an aerobic walking group versus a control group.

The results were dramatic – and are huge for anyone wanting to sidestep dementia and other forms of brain decline.

Adults this age usually lose one to two percent of their hippocampal volume *per year*.

In this study those in the aerobic walking group GAINED an average of 2% in hippocampal volume per year – versus an average 1.4% LOSS for those in the control group!

Now that's what I call teaching an "old dog" new tricks.

And, the aerobic walking group showed marked improvements in memory, too. This is remarkable because the researchers found measurable proof in both the physical organ – the hippocampus – and the mental performance on tests.

This study, published in the *Proceedings of the National Academy of Sciences,* expands on a previous extensive Italian study published in 2008.

The Italian study followed a group of age 65+ adults for four years. They used cognitive assessment tests to determine participants' mental health and then looked for relationships between those and the participants' exercise patterns.

Not only did this study find a staggering 73% *decrease* in dementia for the regular exercisers compared to those who didn't exercise… it also showed that *the intensity of exercise had hardly any bearing on the results.* Walking, climbing stairs, and gardening were just as effective in preventing dementia as more strenuous activities.

As I said, you don't have to be an exercise fanatic to reap the benefits.

It even helped those who already had Alzheimer's

Another study found that those diagnosed with early Alzheimer's who were less fit had *four times more* brain shrinkage compared to more physically fit older adults… suggesting that physical fitness can slow down progression of the disease.

At least two large studies have found a significantly lowered dementia risk in those who had higher physical fitness levels or who exercise three or more times per week.

It's never too late to start. . . but watch out if you quit!

So, you made a New Year's Resolution to exercise more in 2013… And you've already dropped the ball and stashed the gym stuff in the depths of your closet like millions of others.

Did that short-term commitment help you or hurt you?

While there's plenty of evidence to show that you gain benefits from taking up exercise late in life even if you've always been a couch potato… there's also emerging evidence to show you might be wasting your energy if you don't stick with it.

A study presented at the 2012 annual meeting of the Society for Neuroscience in New Orleans showed some troubling results. But the study also pointed to an obvious work-around.

Researchers from the University of Sao Paulo, Brazil took a group of healthy adult rats and let them run as much as they wanted on wheels, which they enjoy doing. The rats were also injected with a substance that measures newly created neurons in the hippocampus, because exercise is known to spark the creation of two to three times as many new hippocampal neurons.

On the other hand, the control group had no running wheels. Both groups were monitored for new brain cell growth.

At the end of the first week, the runners' wheels were locked so they also became inactive.

At the end of week 2, the researchers memory-tested both the exercised and control rats by requiring them to find and remember the location of a platform placed along the wall of a small swimming pool. Rats are not fond of water, so they're motivated to find this escape route. Those with better memories paddled to the platform more easily.

At the end of the second week – the week of no exercise – the rats that had been allowed to run during the first week were much faster on the water test than the controls that had never exercised during the whole two weeks. The exercisers also had two or more times the number of new neurons.

The remaining animals took the same memory test after three weeks or six weeks of inactivity.

The animals that were inactive for three or six weeks performed *FAR* worse on the water maze test than the ones who were only inactive for one week. In other words, performance on the memory test declined with every week of inactivity.

In fact, their memories were about equal to the control animals, the ones that had never exercised. The results suggest how transient your exercise-induced benefits may be.

Brain benefits of exercise are lost quickly

A second study presented at the same conference looked at mood and stress in sedentary animals following several months of running.

They found that after 10 weeks of running, followed by three weeks of inactivity, the running rats' brains were *nearly indistinguishable from those of animals that never exercised. It was as if they'd never run.*

Though these are animal studies, indirect evidence suggests that people are just as vulnerable to losing brain function once regular exercise is stopped.

So it might be wise to stick to that New Year's exercise resolution after all.

Exercise for your brain, not just your body

Remember how "mission critical" your brain is to all of your life? Give it a workout today.

The easiest way to keep your brain sharp is to find some kind of physical activity you love doing, mix it up with an alternative type exercise… then mark it on your calendar as an important appointment.

Because it could prove to be the most important one of your day!

Exercising in the morning before work not only spikes brain activity and prepares it for the day's challenges… it also increases retention of new information and aids problem solving on complex issues.

Many experts also advocate that a morning schedule promotes *regular* workouts, as fewer activities clamor for your attention early in the day.

Looking to change up your workout? Try an activity that requires coordination along with cardio exertion, like a dance class.

If you like crunching time at the gym alone, try circuit workouts, which spike your heart rate while constantly redirecting your attention.

Any way you do it, always remember this doctor's admonition… ***"Exercise is really for the brain, not the body."***

So what have you done today for YOUR brain?

RESOURCES AND FURTHER READING:

http://www.brainrules.net/exercise

Proc Natl Acad Sci U S A. 2004 Jun 1;101(22):8473-8. Epub 2004 May 24. **Voluntary exercise increases axonal regeneration from sensory neurons**. Molteni R, Zheng JQ, Ying Z, Gómez-Pinilla F, Twiss JL. Department of Neurosurgery, University of California, Los Angeles, CA 90095, USA.

http://www.webmd.com/fitness-exercise/features/train-your-brain-with-exercise

http://www.ncbi.nlm.nih.gov/pubmed/15769301

A. J. Gow, M. E. Bastin, S. Munoz Maniega, M. C. Valdes Hernandez, Z. Morris, C. Murray, N. A. Royle, J. M. Starr, I. J. Deary, J. M. Wardlaw. **Neuroprotective lifestyles and the aging brain: Activity, atrophy, and white matter integrity**. *Neurology*, 2012; 79 (17): 1802 DOI: 10.1212/WNL.0b013e3182703fd2

http://www.naturalnews.com/031394_exercise_brain_volume.html

Burns, J.M. et al. 2008. Cardiorespiratory fitness and brain atrophy in early Alzheimer disease. *Neurology, 71*, 210-216

Wang, L., Larson, E.B., Bowen, J.D. & van Belle, G. 2006. Performance-Based Physical Function and Future Dementia in Older People. *Archives of Internal Medicine, 166*, 1115-1120.

Larson, E.B., Wang, L., Bowen, J.D., McCormick, W.C., Teri, L., Crane, P., & Kukull, W. 2006. Exercise Is Associated with Reduced Risk for Incident Dementia among Persons 65 Years of Age and Older. *Annals of Internal Medicine, 144 (2)*, 73-81.

http://well.blogs.nytimes.com/2013/01/09/to-keep-the-brain-benefits-of-exercise-keep-exercising/

Chapter Five

Tone Your Brain
Just Like a Muscle

The same way a light bulb needs electricity to produce light... the brain needs the right amount of stimulation to stay active and keep cognitive abilities sharp.

From the moment you wake up, your brain begins to generate anywhere from 10 to 23 watts of power. That's equal to the amount of energy used to power the average light bulb.

Likewise, regular mental stimulation on a daily basis is critical if you want to enjoy optimum brain health and prevent brain-related diseases. Such stimulation is associated with a decreased risk for Alzheimer's as well as a reduction in the lesions that develop in the brains of people already diagnosed with the disease.

As you get older, cognitive decline becomes a much higher risk that demands attention. According to The Franklin Institute, mental stimulation derived from cognitive brain exercises works to protect the brain from decline.

What's really great about cognitive exercises is that, for the most part, they are cheap… safe… and quick. Mental exercise is an easy, reliable way to get your memory and other essential cognitive abilities back on track and working at their most efficient levels.

There are several forms of cognitive exercises you can try to give your mind the daily workout it needs to keep active and sharp:

Switch to Your Less Dominant Hand

When you use your dominant hand or foot in daily activities it does not require as much brainpower. The brain naturally opts to perform various tasks using your dominant hand or foot because it's the most comfortable option. Basically, the brain is in the habit of going with the dominant choice in the majority of situations.

So when you make the conscious choice to use your less dominant hand or foot, it forces brain cells to learn a new behavior. This strengthens the existing connections between neurons and stimulates the creation of new connections, which help keep the brain engaged and functioning with a renewed sense of youthful energy.

Here are some routine, daily activities where you have the opportunity to switch to your less dominant hand or foot:

- Brushing your teeth

- Combing your hair

- Dialing phone numbers

- Operating a remote control

- Sports activities

- Writing

It may feel awkward at first, but performing such workouts every day will be beneficial in the long run in keeping your mind sharp, active, and focused.

Learning Activities

Learning something completely new and unfamiliar requires a high level of concentration and brainpower. If you don't have a hobby, now is the time to look into getting one because new hobbies help promote improved focus and alertness.

Here are some examples of learning activities that stimulate the brain and increase cognitive activity:

- Brain teasers

- Building models

- Cooking

- Dance, yoga or tai chi classes

- Learning a foreign language

- Photography

- Playing a musical instrument

- Scrapbooking

- Sculpting

The more you learn, the more your brain is required to tap into your memory, thinking skills, and other cognitive resources to allow you to understand and correctly perform the tasks your hobby or course of study require.

People who continue with learning exercises as they enter their senior years can keep their minds sharper than those who do not engage in new interests or activities.

Break Up Your Routines

How many times have you gotten in a car, driven to a friend's house… work… or grocery store and actually paid attention to how you got there?

Over time, when you do a task on a routine basis it requires less and less use of your mental faculties. It's as if the brain goes into autopilot mode and engages only enough to achieve what you need – which is to arrive at your destination, if the task is driving.

As you get older, though, the habit of not being fully engaged and attentive becomes ever more dangerous. Your attention span begins to steadily decrease, putting you at greater risk for distraction and loss of the ability to focus and concentrate.

So to promote more efficient cognitive activity, you can rearrange the furniture in your home… reorganize your office or workplace… or change the routes you take get to various destinations, such as work or the supermarket.

Multi-tasking also works well in keeping brain activity busy and engaged. Monitoring several activities at once and switching nimbly back and forth between them targets weak areas in the mind. It will strengthen them again so they can remain active for the long term.

For example, while exercising you can listen to an audio book or a short story. These two activities stimulate brain activity and work to promote better cognitive engagement because the brain has to maintain attention to follow the story.

Breaking your normal routine can be a fun way to sharpen your mind and gain more years to experience life, while enjoying better brain health.

Internet Searches or Googling

You've probably noticed that technology has become very advanced in almost every area of life. Just about every person in the United States has access to a computer and the Internet. A smart phone you can hold in your hand is a more powerful computer than mainframes of 30 years ago.

These new technology tools give you an opportunity to strengthen key aspects of brain function related to decision-making and complex reasoning skills.

A team of UCLA scientists conducted a series of studies on Internet searching (i.e. "Googling") and the effects it has on the brain. Scientists discovered performing Internet searches requires the use of neural circuitry that is not typically active during other leisure activities such as reading. This increase in neural activity was specifically seen in people who were not first time Internet users.

According to the MRI tests administered during the studies, participants who engaged in regular Internet searchers or Googling had three times the brain activity of first time users.

This study lends weight to a fascinating possibility: Repeated Internet searches may build up cognitive strength and abilities over time, with long-term benefits.

To make effective use of this new form of mental exercise, try spending 15-20 minutes several times during a week Googling different topics on the Internet that you're interested in learning more about. This exercise can be fun because you have the freedom to research anything that interests you, all the while gaining more knowledge and brain strength as you process the incoming information.

Taking advantage of all these safe and easy cognitive exercises along with maintaining a regular physical exercise routine will help you maintain a healthy and strong brain.

Physical exercise keeps the brain in good overall shape, while cognitive exercises keep the mind and cognitive faculties toned. Both forms of exercise are equally important. Incorporate both types of exercise into your daily life so you can reap the maximum benefits for your brain.

RESOURCES AND FURTHER READING:

http://well.blogs.nytimes.com/2011/11/30/how-exercise-benefits-the-brain/

http://www.webmd.com/fitness-exercise/features/train-your-brain-with-exercise

http://www.nytimes.com/2012/04/22/magazine/how-exercise-could-lead-to-a-better-brain.html?pagewanted=all

http://www.prevention.com/health/brain-games/surprising-tips-boost-your-brain/1-google-often

http://www.prevention.com/health/brain-games/surprising-tips-boost-your-brain/2-work-up-sweat

http://www.livestrong.com/article/156760-cognitive-brain-exercises/#ixzz2EO0xJzWz

Chapter Six

The Biggest Risk Factors
for Dementia and Alzheimer's Disease

According to the "2011 Alzheimer's Disease Facts and Figures," published by the Alzheimer's Association, 5.4 million Americans suffer from the debilitating effects of this illness.

Future projections show that by the year 2050 an estimated 16 million Americans – roughly one in four seniors – will be diagnosed with Alzheimer's disease. This is sobering news – a national health disaster. Now is the time to take action to preserve your mind and memories, long before any symptoms appear.

Dementia is one of the fastest growing diseases as well. While Alzheimer's is the major and most frightening cause of dementia, not all dementia is caused by Alzheimer's. As many as half of all cases diagnosed as Alzheimer's disease are actually other forms of dementia – they're not cases of Alzheimer's disease at all.

An estimated 24 million today are living with some form of dementia and – just as with Alzheimer's disease – that number will double – potentially even triple – 20 years down the road.

As Alzheimer's, dementia and other brain diseases are becoming an epidemic, scientists are urgently trying to identify and assess the risk factors that are associated with these diseases and may cause them. If we know the factors that probably cause Alzheimer's and dementia, we can take action to avoid them.

Both dementia and Alzheimer's disease have a variety of risk factors ranging from genetic predispositions to nutritional imbalances or deficiencies.

The gradual loss of mental faculties is the most familiar symptom. This usually starts after age 65, but symptoms can appear much earlier, especially among people who are in the greatest danger as indicated by the risk factors.

On average, the remaining lifespan of people with dementia and Alzheimer's is seven years after the disease begins. And sadly, fewer than five percent – one out of twenty – live longer than 14 years after being diagnosed with their condition.

The most common symptoms linked to dementia and Alzheimer's disease include:

• Aggression

• Confusion

- Difficulty controlling bodily functions

- Loss of long-term and short-term memory

- Loss of language ability

- Mood swings

The progression of Alzheimer's and dementia forces a once active, independent person to become completely dependent on others for even the most basic, trivial needs. The rapid deterioration of memory function… gradual decline in physical activity… and frequent displays of apathetic moods eventually destroy the victim's quality of life.

To lower your risk of Alzheimer's disease and dementia, learn how to reduce the various risk factors that make a person more susceptible.

Once you know these factors and what to do about them, you will no longer feel you can't do anything about brain decline. You'll be able to take a much stronger, proactive approach to protect the health of your brain once you know the potential triggers for brain illness.

Many people believe these diseases are mainly caused by the genes. They think the diseases are hereditary. But Alzheimer's disease and dementia have more complex causes. Poor nutrition may be a bigger factor than genes in determining whether a person will develop these diseases.

In fact, genetic risk factors linked to cognitive decline can remain dormant if a person eats the proper nutrients. So making good nutritional choices has to be a high priority if you aim to reduce your risk of cognitive decline.

Here are some surprising risk factors linked to Alzheimer's disease and dementia…

Excessive Levels of Iron

There's an old saying that goes: "Too much of a good thing can make you sick" and this definitely holds true when it comes to iron in your diet.

True, the body needs iron to support a variety of essential functions. As an example, proteins and enzymes use iron to regulate cell growth and differentiation as well as to transport oxygen throughout the body.

In fact, there's one specific protein in red blood cells that requires a constant supply of iron in order to perform its job properly. That protein is hemoglobin.

Hemoglobin binds to oxygen in the air we breathe, and transports it from the lungs to the tissues. If this process is restricted or slowed down in any way, it results in oxygen deficiency. It's because of hemoglobin that blood is red.

Red blood cells that do not have enough oxygen will quickly begin to die off. As a result, tissues, muscles and other vital organs become malnourished and will start to break down.

Studies show iron deficiency – also known as anemia – is at the top of the list of nutritional deficiencies that affect people in the United States. The most common symptoms associated with low iron levels are fatigue and decreased immune function. If untreated, anemia can lead to serious health problems.

In order to prevent iron deficiency, many people opt for taking an iron supplement. However, even though the body does requires iron for a variety of different functions, too much iron can be toxic for the brain.

How so?

Well, problems arise when there is an accumulation of iron in the blood. Your body needs just enough iron to satisfy the demands of hemoglobin so it can oxygenate cells. Abnormally high iron levels, above this basic need, are not desirable.

Since iron is a very potent oxidizer it can cause serious damage to body tissues, contributing to health problems and diseases like Alzheimer's. To understand what oxidation does, just consider that rust is what happens to iron when it oxidizes. Similarly, oxidation can destroy body tissues.

Your body has a hard time excreting excess iron. Instead, excess iron builds up or accumulates in your organs and tissues. When this happens, dangerous free radicals are produced at an increased rate, posing a serious threat to the health of your brain.

Free radicals are unstable organic molecules that try to bond with other healthy molecules. In the process of doing so, they destroy the health and integrity of these once healthy molecules. The damage escalates as free radicals continue searching for other molecules to bond with. Free radicals have been proven to trigger:

- Aging

- Serious diseases

- Tissue damage

So how does all this relate to preventing brain diseases like Alzheimer's and dementia? Recent studies indicate excessive iron levels are a risk factor for Alzheimer's disease.

When it comes to the brain, free radicals target and attack healthy brain cells and neurons, causing serious damage by slowing down brain signals to the rest of the body.

This leaves the brain trying to use weakened neurons to meet the demands of cognitive function. If neurons aren't healthy, it's virtually guaranteed you'll have greater difficulty with your memory… thinking ability… and problem solving skills.

It's also interesting to point out that studies on brain neurons reveal those with higher traces of iron will be more likely to experience rapid degeneration.

Besides increasing the production of free radicals, another danger posed by high iron levels is that iron is related to the amount of plaque present in the brain's arteries.

People suffering from Alzheimer's usually have high amounts of beta-amyloid plaque in their brains. Iron is extremely reactive with this particular type of plaque and as a result can put you at greater risk for developing Alzheimer's, memory problems, and even stroke.

A breakthrough animal study revealed that simply reducing the amount of iron in the bloodstream also reduced beta-amyloid levels and the levels of the protein phosphotylated tau –both of which are responsible for interrupting the electrical signals between neurons. When iron levels fell, so did levels of these two substances known to be associated with Alzheimer's.

 Researchers also found that when they reduced the amount of excess iron in mice with early stage Alzheimer's, the symptoms associated with the disease became less frequent and severe.

Experts on metal metabolism have conducted numerous studies on the nature of iron and have discovered that metal ions actually play a role in whether or not a person develops Alzheimer's disease. That's why medical professionals and scientists are leaning towards using iron tests to detect Alzheimer's at the earliest stage possible.

It's very interesting to note these studies show iron has a strong tendency to accumulate in areas of the brain associated with memory and thought processes. These are the same two areas that gradually lose function as a result of Alzheimer's disease.

Making it a point to regularly check iron levels should be a part of your preventative healthcare screenings. A simple blood test that measures the level of ferritin in the blood can help identify if iron levels are starting to become imbalanced.

Healthy iron levels reportedly range between 20-80 ng/ml. But the ideal level of iron should stay between 40-60 ng/ml. Iron levels less than 20 ng/ml are a strong indication of iron deficiency, putting you at risk of anemia. Levels higher than 80 ng/ml put you at greater risk for excess iron accumulation and possibly Alzheimer's disease or dementia. Iron levels that reach over 300 ng/ml pose a serious danger for iron toxicity and can eventually lead to long-term, irreversible damage.

Clearly, then, it's safe to say too much iron in the brain creates a toxic environment that can negatively effect overall function and health. So if you're at risk for or currently have high iron levels, it's not too late to take steps to naturally lower them to a much safer level.

Obviously, iron supplements and multivitamin or mineral supplements containing iron should be discontinued (you can easily find multis that don't contain iron). Red meat is also iron-rich and should be cut back or stopped until iron levels are reduced to a safe level. Eat chicken or fish instead.

Certain foods, herbs and spices including green tea and rosemary contain phenolic properties known for reducing iron absorption. Phenolic compounds are normally required for growth and reproduction. They also are full of potent antioxidants. According to Dr. Ray Sahelian, M.D., foods containing phenolic nutrients can increase overall wellness… improve the immune system… and help keep iron levels in check.

The spice curcumin has also proven to be beneficial in naturally lowering iron levels. According to mice studies, curcumin works as an iron chelator that aids the body in the safe and natural elimination of excess iron.

These studies show that mice fed supplemental curcumin experienced a decline in liver ferritin levels. Ferritin is a protein that stores iron so the body can use it later. However, it can also cause too much iron to accumulate over time if not monitored properly.

If your iron levels are too high, the sooner you lower them, the better your chances will be to stop the damage they trigger in the brain.

Low Magnesium Levels

Over 300 cellular metabolic functions require critical amounts of the mineral magnesium. 80 percent of the magnesium needed by the body goes to the cells, where it acts as a catalyst and synthesizing agent. Organs and tissues require plenty of magnesium to keep their functions in good working order.

For years scientists have paid attention to all the vital uses of magnesium within the body. It's widely known as being one of the three or four most essential minerals the body needs for good health.

Common symptoms of magnesium deficiency are muscular tension, irritability, and fatigue. These same symptoms can be linked to many other health problems, so a blood test is required to accurately diagnose magnesium deficiency.

Checking magnesium levels is very important because long-term magnesium deficiency has been linked to a host of health issues including an increased risk of fatal disease. And now, recent studies show magnesium is one of the nutrients the brain requires to prevent Alzheimer's and dementia.

Unfortunately, the majority of people today suffer from magnesium deficiency without even realizing it. Steady depletion of magnesium is associated with advancing age – especially depletion from brain cells. The problem is serious because the brain requires twice the amount of recommended magnesium in order to successfully enhance memory function… preserve brain health… and reach optimum brain activity.

In one Chinese study, conducted at Tsinghua University in Beijing, researchers discovered that magnesium dramatically improved brain health. Researchers believe higher magnesium levels could be a key nutrient in supporting enhanced cognitive function –especially for seniors most at risk for Alzheimer's disease and dementia.

This study showed magnesium has a positive effect on the synaptic plasticity of brain cells. Synaptic plasticity is what enables the brain to make changes… handle stress… maintain stable nerve structure… and recover from trauma. In order for brain cells to maintain this feature they must stay well nourished and properly energized.

Choosing to supplement with magnesium helps ensure the brain is getting the amount it needs to improve overall function. However, not just any form of magnesium will work to increase the levels in brain cells. A specific type of magnesium has the ability to cross into the brain.

According to a 2010 animal model study conducted by MIT researchers, the only form of magnesium that has proven effective in entering into the brain by crossing through the blood-brain barrier was magnesium L-Threonate.

When the mice in this study were administered high doses of magnesium L-Threonate, not only did the magnesium L-Threonate increase the amount of magnesium in brain cells – it also caused measurable benefits in cognitive activity in the test subjects.

Scientists have found magnesium L-Threonate aids neurons by sustaining a healthy balance of activity where they are neither under-stimulated nor over-stimulated. In a sense, it works to make sure all aspects of the brain are functioning at the optimum point. The benefits showed continuous improvement over the long term.

Researchers believe magnesium L-Threonate has the potential to revolutionize what is known about brain malnourishment and ultimately help people achieve and keep optimum cognitive function, even if they've started to experience brain decline.

With the support of magnesium, the brain can meet the cognitive demands required of it without getting stressed or fatigued. Healthy levels of magnesium lead to improvements in:

- Decision making
- Learning
- Memory recall
- Spatial recognition

The most accepted dietary recommendation for magnesium is 400 mg per day. However, a growing number of nutritionists are starting to suggest up to 1000 mg are needed for optimum brain health.

Adding magnesium by means of whole foods will help you reach your daily intake target. Organic green vegetables can provide a substantial amount of the magnesium needed. Experts believe organic green vegetables contain ten times the amount of magnesium found in non-organic vegetables.

Unprocessed sea salt is also high in magnesium. Sea salt is different from the common table salt most people use as a seasoning. In fact, some nutritionists claim table salt, as well as refined sugar and bleached flour, actually deplete magnesium from the body and brain. At any rate, common table salt contains no magnesium while some brands of sea salt are rich in it.

Magnesium is a vital nutrient needed to preserve your mind and brain health for decades to come. Ask your doctor to monitor your levels in order to prevent deficiency from turning your brain into a sitting duck for Alzheimer's and dementia.

Beware of Statins and Anticholinergic Drugs

Two types of drugs pose a serious risk to your brain health and increase your brain's vulnerability to both Alzheimer's disease and dementia – especially when taken on a regular basis:

Anticholinergic drugs – Inhibit the actions of the neurotransmitter acetylcholine to stop the transmission of certain nerve impulses that cause spasms in smooth muscles.

Some examples of these drugs include:

- Antidepressants
- Antihistamines
- Incontinence medications
- Narcotic pain relievers
- Nighttime pain relievers
- Sleep medications

Statin drugs – Commonly prescribed to treat high cholesterol and lower the risk of cardiovascular disease and events from cardiac episodes.

The most popular statin drugs include:

- Atorvastatin (Lipitor)

- Fluvastatin (Lescol)

- Lovastatin (Mevacor)

- Pitavastatin (Livalo)

- Pravastatin (Pravachol)

- Rosuvastatin (Crestor)

- Simvastatin (Zocor)

Both anticholinergic and statin drugs block the production of the brain neurotransmitter acetylcholine. A low presence of acetylcholine in the brain has been found in persons suffering from dementia. It follows that taking these drugs probably increases the risk for dementia.

One study even showed people taking anticholinergic drugs were four times more likely to have higher cognitive impairment than those not taking them. Other studies reveal people who regularly take two of these drugs have an *even higher* risk for cognitive problems.

The side effects posed by statin drugs are an even greater threat to the brain. For starters, these drugs eliminate the brain's supply of coenzyme Q10 (CoQ10) and neurotransmitter precursors.

CoQ10 is another protective nutrient the brain needs in large quantities. It fights free radical damage while working to enhance metabolic energy levels in brain cells.

More importantly, studies show CoQ10 is proving to be a valuable resource in slowing down the progression of Alzheimer's disease…

When scientists administered CoQ10 to both middle-aged and elderly rats they found significant results.

In general, there was a 10 to 40 percent increase in the amount of CoQ10 present in the cerebral cortex of the subject's brains. This rapid increase of CoQ10 in the brain was enough to completely restore levels equivalent to those present in the brains of younger rats.

Two months later, after continuing with the same amount of CoQ10 supplementation, the subjects were tested again and scientists found yet another benefit – the rats had a 29 percent increase in mitochondrial energy. The mitochondria are a cell's "energy factories."

A study presented by Duke University Medical Center added further support by showing the unique properties of CoQ10 not only improve quality of life and life expectancy in people suffering from Alzheimer's disease, but also inhibit the progression of the disease and frequency of its symptoms.

Scientists believe the neuroprotective properties of CoQ10 provide enough positive benefits to warrant its use to treat neurological issues like Alzheimer's disease.

So if statin drugs pose the risk of depleting the brain's supply of CoQ10, then you open yourself up to the risk of severe cognitive decline by taking them on a regular basis.

Statin drugs pose other risks too…

They prevent fat-soluble antioxidants and essential fatty acids – like omega-3s – from reaching the brain to keep it protected, energized, and well nourished. Statins inhibit the production of a biomolecule called low-density lipoprotein, which is critical in transporting essential fatty acids to the brain.

If you currently suffer from high cholesterol or another type of cardiovascular issue and have been taking statin drugs, talk with your doctor about healthier alternatives to these medications so you can prevent long-term damage to your brain health.

Avoid Eating Foods High in Fructose

Sugar is an essential nutrient the brain needs for energy. However, not all types of sugar are good for the brain. Eating foods containing "bad" sugars can significantly affect brain health.

One type of sugar is at the top of the list of ones to avoid – fructose.

This is the type of sugar used to create high-fructose corn syrup – a major ingredient in the following foods (and many others):

• Sodas

• Packaged cookies and pastries

• Condiments

• Sauces

Fructose is classified as a simple sugar – or monosaccharide – that the body can use to create energy for cells. At one point it was believed fructose was a safer alternative to table sugar (sucrose, generally made from sugar cane) because it had a low glycemic index. Foods with low glycemic indexes do not drastically increase blood sugar levels and trigger dangerous imbalances.

Now health advocates have gone to the opposite extreme and often say sucrose is safer than fructose. This belief is mistaken. Both sucrose and fructose are equally dangerous and you should avoid both.

Both the sucrose and high-fructose corn syrup molecules are essentially half glucose (the healthy sugar) and half fructose (the dangerous sugar). So you do not avoid the dangers of fructose by eating sucrose or cane sugar. The body breaks both of them down into glucose (good) and fructose (bad).

Nutritional experts from the American Diabetes Association published studies showing that high levels of fructose can overwhelm the body's natural ability to process this sugar safely. As a result, natural functions in the body are interrupted, causing complete chaos – and the brain is not immune to these effects.

Fructose is toxic for the brain. How so?

For starters, the brain reacts in a completely different way to fructose than it does to glucose. The body manufactures glucose itself from carbohydrates like wheat, fat or potatoes. Glucose naturally circulates in your blood and, in moderate amounts, it's essential to good health.

Nine participants in one study were administered either fructose… glucose… or a saline (salt) control to determine how the brain metabolizes the two sugars. Researchers then administered brain scans specifically monitoring the brain's hypothalamus area.

The results showed glucose significantly increased neural activity while fructose *lowered* **neural activity.** So fructose can be considered a brain hazard.

Fructose also prevents the liver from making cholesterol. This is a serious issue for the brain because 25 percent of the cholesterol in the body is found in the brain. Too much fructose in the body distracts the liver from its more important job of making cholesterol. Instead, trying to process fructose becomes the liver's primary focus.

Cholesterol is essential in the activity of neurons. Poor neuron activity increases your risk of impaired memory and dementia. Clearly then, cholesterol is a critical building block for maintaining healthy brain activity. Having just the right amount can make the difference between poor and optimum brain function.

Fructose is also a proven link to altering the brain's craving mechanism. When you eat fructose, the brain doesn't receive the signal that you've had something to eat, and you continue to be hungry. What's more, fructose causes serious damage to both the circulatory and nervous systems.

In conducting a study on the effects of sugar on the brain published in the *Journal of Physiology*, researchers from UCLA's David Geffen School of Medicine specifically explored the changes fructose causes in the brain activity of rats…

For five days, twice a day, researchers trained all the rats in the study to complete a complicated maze. Once the maze was successfully memorized, the rats were split into separate groups.

Both groups received a solution of high-fructose corn syrup instead of water. However, one of the groups was also given a combination of two powerful nutrients containing omega-3 fatty acids.

After 6 weeks, the maze test was administered to the rats again. Researchers discovered the rats that received only high-fructose corn syrup struggled with memory recall and experienced a slower rate in problem solving. High-fructose corn syrup made them stupid.

The rats in the other group that were given omega-3 fatty acids in addition to the high-fructose corn syrup had a faster completion rate of the maze.

This study highlights the dangers of a long-term diet high in fructose. It will ultimately alter the brain's ability to learn and recall information and increases the risk of memory loss. It undermines these critical components of strong cognitive function. It very likely puts you at greater risk for Alzheimer's… dementia… and other brain diseases.

This same study also showed the power of omega-3 fatty acids in combating the cognitive decline that results from fructose. The fatty acids helped protect the brain from damage despite the amount of fructose present.

Here's another scary thing about fructose that shows just how much it can threaten brain health…

About 10 percent of today's modern diet comes from foods containing fructose. Recent estimates show the average American consumes over 40 pounds of high-fructose corn syrup each year – that's about 300 percent more than the dietary recommended amount!

So to protect your brain from being an open target for the dangerous effects of fructose, make an effort to consume less than 25 grams daily. That's a little more than one ounce.

Taking a proactive approach and reducing these risk factors will help keep your mind healthy, quick and alert for years to come.

RESOURCES AND FURTHER READING:

http://www.alz.org/downloads/facts_figures_2011.pdf

http://lowcarbdiets.about.com/od/nutrition/a/fructosedangers.htm

http://articles.mercola.com/sites/articles/archive/2011/02/28/new-study-confirms-fructose-affects-your-brain-very-differently-than-glucose.aspx

http://www.huffingtonpost.com/2012/05/16/sugar-makes-you-stupid-ucla_n_1521812.html

http://www.fitsugar.com/High-Fructose-Corn-Syrups-Effect-Brain-23134099

http://www.swansonvitamins.com/health-library/products/magnesium-l-threonate-brain-function-mental-health-support.html

http://www.naturalnews.com/028171_magnesium_brain_function.html#ixzz2E2QjhmR7

http://www.empr.com/medications-with-significant-anticholinergic-properties/article/123667/#

http://www.thoracic.org/clinical/copd-guidelines/for-patients/what-kind-of-medications-are-there-for-copd/what-are-anticholinergic-medications.php

http://www.drugs.com/drug-class/anticholinergics-antispasmodics.html

http://heartdisease.about.com/cs/cholesterol/a/statins.htm

http://www.disabled-world.com/health/aging/dementia/statistics.php#ixzz2E2KYjl6s

http://articles.mercola.com/sites/articles/archive/2012/07/19/excess-iron-leads-to-alzheimers.aspx?e_cid=20120719_DNL_artNew_1#_edn1

http://www.disabled-world.com/health/aging/dementia/statistics.php

http://www.smartbodyz.com/CoQ10Text.htm

http://www.livestrong.com/article/429201-coenzyme-q10-in-alzheimers/#ixzz2EQ3btKRA

http://articles.mercola.com/sites/articles/archive/2012/07/19/excess-iron-leads-to-alzheimers.aspx?e_cid=20120719_DNL_artNew_1

http://www.cdc.gov/nutrition/everyone/basics/vitamins/iron.html

http://www.livestrong.com/article/81861-list-foods-phenolic-compounds/#ixzz2E20KFaCy

http://www.nlm.nih.gov/medlineplus/ency/article/003490.htm

Chapter Seven

The Common Brain Destroyer Nobody Knows About

Unknown to most people and most doctors, there's a common food that can destroy your brain and make you suffer dementia as devastating as Alzheimer's. Chances are, you eat this food every day and if you started losing your memory and personality you'd never even suspect this food was to blame.

The everyday food that's so potentially dangerous? Bread.

Do you ever give any thought to the fact that what you eat at every meal can have serious, unexpected consequences for the health of your brain? You should. Something as seemingly harmless as a piece of bread can knock out pieces of your memory or destroy it entirely.

Consider the case of a 58-year-old who thought he was suffering from Alzheimer's disease. He began forgetting conversations minutes after they ended. (He didn't just forget the subjects of those conversations, he forgot he'd ever had them.) He would hit the gas pedal instead of the brakes on his car. He'd tell his friends the same story he'd just told them a couple of minutes before. He couldn't even remember where the silverware was kept in a house where he'd lived for twenty years.

And just when he thought he might soon be put in an institution, he heard about a study at the Mayo Clinic that showed some people can suffer from Alzheimer's-like symptoms if they're sensitive to gluten, a group of proteins found in wheat, barley and rye. Of course, in the American diet wheat is by far the most common of these three grains.

Seeing a ray of hope, he decided to try a gluten-free diet. He figured he had nothing to lose. His doctor couldn't offer him any help. According to the doctor, his type of early-onset dementia was incurable.

So he gave up bread and other foods like beer, cake, pizza and pretzels that contain gluten.

The result? Within two weeks, with that single change of diet, his brain began to mend. His memory began a steady return. His friends and family immediately noticed the difference. The angry, forgetful, confused man had recovered the use of his brain.

Destructive Proteins

Gluten is the conglomeration of proteins that give dough its gooey texture. But in susceptible people, gluten irritates the immune system, leading immune cells to attack the body. These immune cells can damage and destroy nerves and brain cells.

No one knows for sure how many people suffer these consequences. Medical researchers have only begun to get a handle on how many of us are intolerant to the gluten we eat.

The most important facts about gluten include:

- No one can digest gluten. You may tolerate gluten, but it passes through your body without being assimilated and it has no health benefits.

- The best estimate is that 1 percent of Americans suffer from the most serious form of gluten intolerance, known as celiac disease, an autoimmune condition that can destroy the digestive tract, nerves and brain. Celiac disease is extremely serious and can eventually lead to death. Some experts speculate that mild gluten intolerance is actually a moderate form of celiac disease.

- Anywhere from 6 to 20 percent of Americans (and maybe more) suffer what is currently termed "gluten sensitivity." These people haven't been diagnosed with celiac disease but suffer health problems from an immune reaction to gluten. By far the majority of these people don't know they're sick because their systems can't handle gluten. They just suffer from a mystery illness their doctors can't diagnose – such as bad digestion, chronic pain, skin rashes – or loss of memory.

- Research indicates that you can develop celiac disease or gluten sensitivity at any age. You can be OK with gluten today but wake up with celiac disease tomorrow. As you age, your chances of celiac disease grow.

Brain Problems

Gluten's harm to your brain can be devastating. This problem has not received a great deal of attention in the media, but the studies that have looked into this form of brain destruction are disturbing.

For example, when Mayo Clinic researchers investigated 13 people with celiac disease who were developing dementia and other serious cognitive deficits at a relatively young age, their findings clearly pointed toward gluten as the culprit.

These eight women and five men were all plagued by amnesia, confusion and personality changes. In several cases, when researchers put them on a gluten-free diet, their memory loss ceased or was reversed.

Unique Mental Condition

According to Joseph Murray, M.D., the Mayo Clinic gastroenterologist who took part in this study, "There has been a fair amount written before about celiac disease and neurological issues like peripheral neuropathy (nerve problems causing numbness or pain) or balance problems, but this degree of brain problem – the cognitive decline we've found here – has not been recognized before. I was not expecting there would be so many celiac disease patients with cognitive decline."

Dr. Murray points out that an autoimmune reaction to gluten:

• Leads to nutrient deficiencies. When the immune system attacks the intestines, it destroys the villi, the part of the intestinal wall that absorbs nutrients like vitamin E, vitamin B12 and folate.

• Causes an increase in inflammatory cytokines. These immune cells increase inflammation that damage brain tissue.

• Sets off a direct immune attack on brain cells and nerves.

Memory Deficit

Experts estimate that about one in ten people with celiac have brain and neurological problems, although the research on this issue is still sketchy. Along with wiping your memory clean, the attack on nerve cells can cause neuropathies – pain and tingling in the hands, feet and other parts of the body. Sometimes these problems are irreversible. In other cases, going on a gluten-free diet may alleviate the discomfort.

Dr. Murray points out that until now, if you had cognitive impairment and were developing dementia, it was generally considered incurable. "This is key that we may have discovered a reversible form of cognitive impairment," he says.

And William Hu, M.D., Ph.D., who also took part in the Mayo study says, "For patients who come in with atypical forms of dementia, we need to consider checking for celiac disease."

So, if you're having trouble with your memory, trying a gluten-free diet (no foods containing wheat, barley or rye) may help. If gluten is the root of your brain problem, going gluten-free may start improving your brain power within a couple of weeks. It did for the 58-year-old whose doctor told him there was no hope.

RESOURCES AND FURTHER READING:

http://www.niams.nih.gov/Health_Info/Bone/Osteoporosis/Conditions_Behaviors/celiac.asp

http://somvweb.som.umaryland.edu/absolutenm/templates/?a=1474

http://www.livingwithout.com/issues/4_15/qa_augsep11-2554-1.html

http://www.ncbi.nlm.nih.gov/pubmed/?term=celiac+josephs

http://www.ncbi.nlm.nih.gov/pubmed/22538308

Chapter Eight

Stress – The Subtle Brain Destroyer

Neurodegeneration… brain diseases… and impaired cognitive activity become much more of a risk in people who suffer from chronic stress.

The world we live in today subjects us to extreme levels of stress. Many people are worried, under intense pressure, desperately short of time, buried under job and financial problems – and more. It's a long list. As a result, the body is not able to manage the constant flood of negative side effects of stress.

Stress truly lives up to its name of being a silent killer, and your brain is one of its primary targets…

Scientists are realizing more and more just how dangerous chronic stress is for the brain. Both short-term and long-term stress pose risks to the brain.

For starters, stress is directly linked to how well the brain is able to absorb, produce, and utilize the nutrients it needs to maintain healthy activity and good overall cognitive function.

The overall level of stress in your body affects the successful digestion and assimilation of foods containing critical brain nutrients. Poor digestion robs the brain of the energy it needs to operate efficiently.

In 2009 the *American Journal of Clinical Nutrition* published a Norwegian study that reported low choline levels were the result of higher rates of anxiety or stress. As explained in an earlier chapter, choline is the critical component needed to keep communication between the brain's neurons and neurotransmitters sharp and active. Without choline the brain is unable to effectively produce healthy neurotransmitters and communication is significantly impaired.

High levels of stress can even physically alter brain cells, which will then compromise the integrity of brain structure and function.

When it comes to diseases like Alzheimer's, some scientists are making a greater effort to discover more about the powerful role stress plays in brain health…

According to one breakthrough study published in the *Journal of the Federation of American Societies for Experimental Biology*, scientists from the University of Southern California found a strong link between neurodegeneration and stress and how this in turn increases a person's risk for Alzheimer's…

In this study, scientists examined the brains of rats that had been exposed to psychological stress. They found these rats had high activity of the RCAN1 gene. The researchers who conducted the study believe chronic stress causes the over-expression (heightened activity) of RCAN1, putting the organism in serious danger of developing some form of neurodegenerative disease.

In the average healthy adult, the RCAN1 gene is responsible for helping brain cells manage stress in a healthy, safe manner. However, when there is excessive activity of RCAN1 it changes from a helper to a hazard that can cause serious damage to neurons and proteins. It also poses the added risk of obstructing brain signals from reaching their destinations. Lack of brain communication raises the risk for brain disease.

Scientists believe the two leading causes for neurodegeneration associated with Alzheimer's disease are:

- Overproduction of the amyloid beta peptide protein

- Tau hyperphosphorylation – A condition resulting in tau proteins binding together, making it next to impossible for brain signals to travel effectively.

The overproduction of RCAN1 has been identified as a trigger to both these conditions.

With poor brain communication resulting from overproduction of RCAN1, a person can start displaying symptoms linked to Alzheimer's as early as age 40.

Stress is an all-around brain robber. It not only makes life unpleasant, it also jeopardizes your memory and puts you at the mercy of hard-to-control moods. High levels of stress have been proven toxic to the brain.

The sooner you reduce your stress levels – the better the chances will be for your brain to make a full recovery from the long term effects of stress.

ADDITIONAL READING:

http://news.usc.edu/#!/article/28793/Chronic-Stress-Can-Cause-Brain-Disease

Chapter Nine

Could This One Mineral be *The* Secret of Good Brain Health?

In recent years, one mineral has shown outstanding benefits in combating brain disorders. Most people know little or nothing about this mineral, but it could be *the* key nutrient to take your brain health to the next level...

You may know **lithium** as a treatment for certain kinds of mental illness. In the psychiatric world, this metal has produced tremendous success in treating mood disorders and other forms of mental problems.

Studies show lithium works to decrease abnormal brain activity. Doctors have prescribed lithium for decades and proven it's the most potent treatment for a wide variety of mental disorders – even when taken in small doses.

In the United States, lithium is the number one treatment prescribed for bipolar disorder. If untreated, people who are bipolar experience wild swings between two states – mania (characterized by unreasonable happiness and enthusiasm) and depression. Lithium works to prevent mania or manic episodes and relieves depression as well.

While you may wonder how a person can be too full of energy and enthusiasm, bipolar patients can engage in dangerous, erratic behavior during their manic episodes. Exactly the kind of behavior a layperson would call "crazy." And, of course, deep depression is miserable and dangerous for the opposite reason. Lithium moderates the mood swings.

In one study, 10 patients suffering from manic depression or bipolar disorder were given a shot of lithium. All 10 patients experienced significant improvement in their symptoms and were able to return to normal daily activities.

Lithium's well-documented success in treating bipolar disorder has led some doctors to ask if it can offer any help in treating age-related brain diseases. A lot of evidence suggests the answer is a resounding "yes." New findings suggest lithium may be important for treating Alzheimer's and dementia. . .and for helping perfectly healthy people hang on to their memories and their general brain health.

Let's take a look at what the researchers have found. . .

Can Lithium Prevent Alzheimer's Disease and Dementia?

Research has only scratched the surface in investigating the effects of lithium on the brain. But growing evidence supports lithium's ability to improve overall brain health and fight the symptoms related to Alzheimer's disease and dementia.

Lithium's tremendous benefits have stumped scientists because it's a very simple element. You know it as one of the elements in the periodic table, if you've ever taken a chemistry class. It's not a fancy compound or a manufactured drug. In fact, the chemical properties of lithium are very similar to some of those found in common table salt.

On the most basic level, lithium benefits people suffering from mental illness in two ways:

• It protects brain neurons from damage and death.

• It stimulates new nerve cell growth that alleviates existing damage in the brain.

It so happens these same benefits are exactly what the brain needs to combat Alzheimer's disease.

Dr. De-Maw Chuang, a biologist at the National Institute of Mental Health, conducted research to look for the possible benefits lithium could have on the brain.

During one of his first studies, Dr. Chuang saw just how much lithium actually protects brain neurons from damage…

In an *in vitro* (test tube) experiment, Dr. Chuang treated nerve cells using the natural brain chemical called glutamate. Glutamate is absolutely essential for survival and is a primary component in stimulating electric signals in brain neurons. But when present in large amounts, glutamate can be damaging.

The amount of glutamate in the brain can be significantly affected by a number of different things. For example, when the brain experiences trauma or stroke, brain cells die and very high amounts of glutamate are released. When glutamate levels become too high, the death rate of brain cells dramatically increases. This effect is seen in patients suffering from various degenerative conditions.

In Dr. Chuang's lab study, after glutamate was added to the nerve cell lab cultures all the cells were completely destroyed. However, when Dr. Chuang added lithium before adding glutamate the results were drastically different. **All of the cells were almost completely protected from glutamate's damaging effect.** None of the other drugs tested provided benefits that compared to those of lithium.

But these test tube experiments didn't prove whether or not the same results would occur in an actual live brain…

So in another study, Dr. Chuang administered lithium to rat subjects to determine if similar protective characteristics would show. After giving the rats lithium for a few weeks, Dr. Chuang next triggered strokes in the rats by artificially blocking a brain artery. The results were impressive…

The rats taking lithium experienced only half as much brain damage as the rats in the control group that did not receive lithium. Rats in the lithium group also experienced benefits during the time following the stroke. The results showed lithium continued to prevent the type of degenerative damage normally found in stroke victims.

This benefit is exciting because it means lithium can potentially be the key to saving stroke victims from severe brain damage.

But what about Alzheimer's disease and dementia? Is it possible that lithium can help combat the effects of these diseases on your brain?

According to a 2004 research study conducted at the *Eve Topf and National Parkinson Foundation Centers of Excellence for Neurodegenerative Diseases Research*, when lithium was administered to mice afflicted with Parkinson's disease the same neuro-protective benefits were seen.

Researchers believe lithium can potentially help prevent neuron death in diseases that cause the brain to gradually lose certain functional capabilities. Parkinson's disease and Alzheimer's disease resemble one another in this respect.

During an exploratory study, University of Pennsylvania developmental biologist Peter Klein noticed a promising benefit lithium could provide in the treatment of Alzheimer's disease.

As mentioned in previous chapters, Alzheimer's disease causes two observable abnormalities in the brain structure:

- Amyloid plaques – Hard flat growths.

- Neurofibrillary tangles – Comprised of braided fibers.

Researchers have reported that lithium works to prevent damage caused by beta-amyloid plaque by inhibiting its secretion and blocking existing beta-amyloid protein from causing further damage to healthy brain cells. This effect alone may drastically slow the progression of Alzheimer's disease, because studies indicate the larger the amount of beta-amyloid protein present – the worse Alzheimer's becomes.

In the second abnormality in Alzheimer's, studies show that when the brain protein called tau is over-activated, it increases the risk of neurofibrillary tangles. As a result, neuronal degeneration and general brain damage related to Alzheimer's disease are much higher. Lithium works to stop the progression of these nerve-cell damaging effects.

Here's something else interesting about amyloid plaque and neurofibrillary tangles…

Both these abnormalities involve different factors that trigger the brain to produce them. However, an in-depth study revealed that both neurofibrillary tangles and amyloid plaques have significant traces of the protein GSK-3. This particular protein has been identified as a contributing factor in the development of these two Alzheimer's-related abnormalities.

Peter Klein's study discovered that lithium works to block or suppress the actions of GSK-3 that trigger these brain abnormalities. This offers hope that lithium is an effective preventative treatment for those people most at risk for Alzheimer's disease and dementia.

The long-standing neuroprotective benefits seen in lithium could reduce the number of neurons lost by people suffering from Alzheimer's disease. It may even contribute to cell growth and healthier brain cells.

Other studies add further weight to support the use of lithium therapy to treat Alzheimer's disease…

During 1999 and 2000, three research studies were published out of Wayne State University of Medicine regarding the effects of lithium on Alzheimer's disease. These studies brought to light the interaction between lithium and B-cell lymphoma/leukemia-2 gene or Bc1-2 protein.

To be fully protected against Alzheimer's disease and dementia, the brain needs sufficient levels of the Bc1-2 protein. According to the three Wayne State studies, lithium was the first substance to successfully increase the concentration of Bc1-2 in brain tissue.

Adding further support, these same studies also showed lithium decreased the supply of GSK-2b – a destructive protein known to trigger Alzheimer's disease – in brain tissue.

Lithium also works to combat another possible trigger for Alzheimer's disease – aluminum. While there's a popular belief that aluminum causes Alzheimer's, the evidence is not conclusive. All the same, there's no benefit to having high aluminum levels.

Some studies that examined the brains of Alzheimer's patients found they tend to have excess aluminum. It's best if the body is able to naturally remove unabsorbed or excess amounts. Lithium helps safely chelate excess amounts of aluminum from the body before it has a chance to build-up in the brain. In the chelation process, an element or chemical – in this case, lithium – bonds with the aluminum, lead, mercury or another unwanted metal and the compound is excreted from the body.

It's clear lithium shows tremendous promise when it comes to preventing Alzheimer's disease, but what about other types of dementia? Can this mineral provide any restorative benefits?

According to Dr. Jonathan Wright, M.D., published author, founder of the Tahoma Clinic, member of the medical advisory board for the Life Extension Foundation and avid supporter of lithium-related therapies, even though Alzheimer's disease and non-Alzheimer's dementia are not the same, both affect the brain in similar ways. Dr. Wright firmly believes lithium can help slow or prevent the progression of non-Alzheimer's dementia with the same success seen in people with Alzheimer's disease.

That's why for over 10 years Dr. Wright himself has been supplementing with 20 mg daily of lithium orotate to protect his brain and maintain sharper memory function.

Clearly, there's strong evidence to support the use of lithium to treat brain diseases. But there are even more positive benefits lithium provides for the brain…

Lithium fights brain shrinkage

Mental illnesses and diseases like Alzheimer's and dementia are associated with brain atrophy or shrinkage. When the brain shrinks, nerve cells can no longer communicate effectively with one another. This impairment triggers a host of cognitive complications that affect general brain function.

Lithium may well hold the key to re-establishing healthy connections between damaged nerve cells and restoring the fast-acting synapses that keep cognitive functions sharp…

In studying the brains of patients with bipolar disorder, scientists discovered their frontal lobes – which control cognitive functions – are smaller and have a higher rate of nerve cell degeneration than do those of healthy people. However, in those patients given lithium, scientists took brain scans and found a significant increase in gray matter. The lithium effectively helped combat the brain shrinkage normally seen in patients with bipolar disorder.

Several studies conducted by Wayne State University researchers reported that the gray matter of patients treated with lithium grew by roughly 3 percent. The treatment even helped regenerate brain cells damaged by disease or injury.

In conditions such as Alzheimer's and dementia where nerve cell shrinkage is a specific side effect, lithium went a long way toward correcting the damage.

This effect of lithium suggests the mineral might be an effective means to combat diseases characterized by ongoing brain cell death. The list includes dementia and Alzheimer's.

In 1999, the British medical journal *Lancet* published findings in which just four weeks of high-dose lithium therapy triggered a significant increase in brain volume and the production of billions of healthy new brain cells. Stimulating brain cell growth helps strengthen the overall integrity of the brain and increase its ability to fight off factors known to trigger Alzheimer's and dementia.

This study calls into question the widely accepted belief that a person is born with all the brain cells they will ever have and that brain shrinkage is just an unavoidable part of getting old.

The truth (as already suggested in Chapter 4) is that the brain can generate new cells if given the right support. By taking the initiative in nutrition and exercise, you can maintain an active, youthful, healthy brain.

How Much Lithium Does the Brain Need?

More research is needed (that's almost always the case with nutritional solutions, which receive little support from the medical establishment). But considering all the protective and restorative benefits lithium appears to offer in preventing brain disease and brain loss, it's worthwhile to add it to your diet.

Very few vitamin and mineral supplements contain lithium – despite the amazing benefits it offers. It's necessary to purchase a separate lithium supplement. There are several reputable brands, widely available online without a prescription. They're very inexpensive (eight or ten cents a pill) compared to most supplements. Unfortunately, lithium is seldom available in stores because its benefits are not widely known.

There are two forms of lithium that can be taken as a supplement: *lithium aspartate* and *lithium orotate*.

According to the late Dr. Hans Nieper, a German orthomolecular physician, supplementing with lithium orotate is much more effective because this form is easily transported inside brain cells. This allows for ingesting a much lower dose and reduces the risk for lithium toxicity or overdose. Use these supplements only as directed by the manufacturer. This is NOT a case where "more is always better."

If you do decide to supplement with lithium, please be aware that too much can be toxic, while too little leaves the brain at greater risk of brain aging and disease.

High doses of lithium are usually administered only to persons suffering from some form of mental illness like bipolar disorder or manic depression. For example a person suffering from manic depression would be administered anywhere from 90 to 180 milligrams of lithium in the form of 900 to 1800 milligrams of lithium carbonate. With these high levels a person needs to be

Don't Drink Coffee? You Still Might Be Losing Acetylcholine…

It's not just coffee that threatens the brain's supply of acetylcholine. There are other equally destructive foods that threaten production as well.

Regularly consuming other caffeinated products like sodas, tea and energy drinks or eating a lot of chocolate can inhibit the rate of acetylcholine production and continue the vicious cycle of scavenging and stealing this chemical from other parts of the brain.

The brain's natural supply will eventually become depleted if these beverages and foods continue to upset the balance of this essential brain chemical.

So, to keep your neurotransmitters from being deficient in acetylcholine and turning against your brain, it's advisable to consume these foods in moderation.

under careful medical supervision.

When it comes to a healthy person who wants to protect the brain on a daily basis much lower levels of lithium are adequate.

According to leading experts in brain-lithium interaction, 10 to 20 milligrams of either lithium aspartate or lithium orotate can provide the brain with enough protection to effectively fight diseases and general aging.

As each pill is generally 5 mg, you can start with a much lower dose than 10 or 20 mg, and observe any changes that occur in your body and your mind – good or bad. It would be ideal to do this under a doctor's direction, but unfortunately few doctors know of lithium's potential benefits for healthy people. You're probably not going to get any support from your doctor if you decide to supplement with lithium.

This dosage of 10 to 20 mg has been proven low enough to avoid interfering with other critical functions of the body, yet still provides powerful protective benefits to the brain.

According to Dr. Wright, low-dose lithium is defined as anything up to a maximum of 55 mg of elemental lithium per day. However, 55 mg is actually much higher than OTC lithium makers recommend. It's about the equivalent of one 300 mg capsule of prescription lithium carbonate given to mental patients, or 11 tablets of over the counter lithium aspartate or orotate. Dr. Wright says anything over this amount needs to be monitored with regular blood testing by a doctor to prevent toxicity and organ damage. DO NOT TAKE MORE THAN THE MANUFACTURER RECOMMENDS ON THE BOTTLE.

Healthy Dietary Sources for Lithium

You can also increase the level of lithium in the brain by eating lithium-rich foods. There are a variety of healthy foods containing potent amounts of lithium.

You may be in luck if you happen to live in an area where the soil is rich in lithium (and if you eat locally grown food). Plants readily absorb this mineral, and so do you when you eat the plants.

If your local soil is high in lithium, you may have the local water supply to thank. Studies show that 1 to 10 mcg of lithium occur in surface water and approximately 0.18 mcg/L of lithium is naturally found in seawater. The latter may be relevant if you live in an area that was an ancient seabed.

Your tap water may naturally contain some traces of lithium. However, higher concentrations are found in mineral water – especially if it's sourced from springs. The location where the water is obtained determines the level of lithium concentration present. Unfortunately, the numerous brands of bottled spring water don't provide data on how much lithium they might contain.

It's too bad, because researchers have observed remarkable benefits from drinking lithium-rich water.

A study published in 2011 in the *British Journal of Psychiatry* found that areas with high lithium levels in their groundwater had lower rates of suicide.

Over 20 years ago, researchers from the University of California studied various counties in Texas and measured lithium levels in their water supply. They discovered that people living in counties with the highest concentration of lithium in their water supply had lower rates of suicide and lower rates of mental hospital admissions for neurosis, personality disorders, and psychosis.

These studies suggest, once again, the powerful effect of lithium on the brain. Even in view of the limited science available to us as this is written, it seems likely that the overall brain health of people in these Texas counties probably improved as a result of the steady supply of lithium in their drinking water.

Besides water, you can also get a bit of lithium in food. A study published in the *Journal of the American College of Nutrition* said "vegetables and grains make up anywhere from 66 to 90 percent of the average person's lithium intake." Just keep in mind that for most people, that "average intake" is much too low.

Meat provides a little bit of lithium – it delivers 0.012 mg/kg in a 0.21 kg serving size (about 7.4 ounces). Vegetables and grains give you double that amount of lithium. So vegetables and grains are the best option to consume lithium in your food.

This study indicates that the amount of lithium present "on average" is tiny. . .far less than you'd need to achieve a therapeutic result. Again, keep in mind that the amount of lithium you absorb from foods can vary based on how they were grown and how much lithium was present in the soil.

The best sources of dietary lithium come from the following food groups:

- **Grains** – Trace amounts of lithium can be found in all grains. However, certain grains absorb greater amounts of lithium from the soil than others. According to the *International Journal of Food Sciences and Nutrition*, grains that provide the highest amount of lithium are hulled wheat and emmer.

- **Vegetables** – So called nightshade vegetables – sweet and hot peppers, tomatoes, and eggplant – boast the highest lithium content. Potatoes, cabbage and cauliflower are also high in lithium.

- **Dairy & animal products** – Lithium is found in the primary food sources of dairy cows. After these foods are digested, lithium is present in the milk. Consuming milk and cheese as well as other dairy products delivers significant doses of lithium to the brain. One study reported an intake of 0.44 kg of dairy foods per day (almost a pound) provides you with a lithium content of 0.50 mg/kg. This means a very large amount of dairy products would have to be consumed to achieve a therapeutic dose of lithium.

- **Herbs** – Various herbs are able to absorb healthy amounts of lithium through soil and water. Paprika, marjoram and cinnamon are mentioned as being lithium-rich. The well-known chamomile herb contains ample amounts of lithium and can be safely used in tea. And, of all things, **black tea** is rich in lithium.

Incorporating these food-based lithium sources into your daily diet will help protect brain cells from being destroyed by brain diseases.

A Word of Caution about Lithium...

Studies show absorbing as little as 30 percent more lithium than your body needs can cause serious adverse side effects. It is not likely that a person supplementing with over-the-counter lithium will experience these side effects if the directions for use are followed. Toxicity is not a major worry, but you should be aware that it can happen.

The Best Kept Mineral Secret...

Lithium is truly a miracle mineral. But what's disappointing is how little action is being taken to learn more about lithium therapy and develop it into a first-line resource for brain health.

This may be the reason: If more people realize the extent to which lithium protects brain and nerve cells, the profits of drug and pharmaceutical companies (estimated at more than 64 billion dollars a year) might be affected. Alzheimer's disease and dementia are a growth industry.

Many more millions of people will succumb to these dreadful diseases as our population ages and it becomes more common for people to live into their eighties and nineties. Lithium is incredibly inexpensive and all the evidence points to the likelihood that it could put a big dent in this national health crisis.

Compared to some of the major drugs prescribed for treating Alzheimer's symptoms, a 30-day supply of lithium aspartate would cost only 6 dollars. For that small monthly cost you could transform the health of your brain for decades to come.

Every person is different, and that includes the way we respond to lithium. This is why it's recommended to start low (5 mg of lithium orotate, for example) and only gradually work up to 10 or 20 mg per day.

Persons living in an area where the food and water are already lithium-rich, and who take lithium supplements as well, are perhaps more likely to experience lithium toxicity. The fact is, so few people supplement with lithium, toxic episodes are extremely rare, except for mental patients on prescription lithium.

One way to counteract any possible adverse side effects of lithium is to take fish oil and flaxseed oil either in a supplement or by adding them to your meal plan. Anecdotal evidence suggests that bipolar patients taking very high doses of lithium were able to counter the toxic effects by taking these omega-3-rich oils. For these patients it was essential to remain on high lithium doses to treat their mood disorder, and the oils enabled them to do that. In any case, these natural oils also help promote healthier brain function and are valuable for anyone who wants to promote better health.

The most common side effects associated with lithium toxicity are slight shaking of the hands and fingers… nausea and other flu-like symptoms… and high blood pressure. The literature also mentions protein in the urine as a symptom. If these symptoms appear, stop taking supplemental lithium. If you wish to resume, do so under a doctor's supervision and start with a low dose. A doctor can check your blood for lithium levels. Based on these reports, you should not "self-treat" with lithium if you have high blood pressure. It should be done only under a doctor's supervision.

RESOURCES AND FURTHER READING:

http://www.livestrong.com/article/519437-what-foods-contain-lithium/#ixzz2NG8ozCib

http://www.livestrong.com/article/327470-natural-sources-of-lithium/#ixzz2NBsu3jVi

http://www.ehow.com/facts_5625232_foods-natural-source-lithium.html#page=1

http://discovermagazine.com/2010/the-brain-2/27-metal-marvel-mended-brains-50-years-lithium#.UTd0oI6I-pE

http://rockcreekfreepress.tumblr.com/post/409440581/lithium

http://wrightnewsletter.com/files/2003/08/nah_0308.pdf

http://collectivewizdom.com/Lithium-LithiumRichFoods.html

http://wrightnewsletter.com/files/2003/08/nah_0308.pdf

Chapter Ten

The Dangers of Coffee

Are you a coffee drinker? If you are, what's the reason? Do you drink coffee for the taste… or would it be more accurate to say you rely on it to give you a quick energy boost to start your day?

These are important questions because it's true that coffee does play a role in brain activity. Yet a large majority of people don't realize exactly how strong this interaction is or the potential dangers drinking coffee poses to the health of your brain….

What actually happens to the brain when you drink coffee?

Within seconds of the first sip, the brain begins to produce and release a large quantity of brain chemicals. These are what give you that energy boost or "coffee buzz" that makes you feel good, alert, and ready to take on whatever challenges come your way.

Caffeine plays a strong role in triggering this energy boost. The caffeine in coffee (and other caffeinated beverages such as tea and colas) blocks the brain chemical known as adenosine. This particular brain chemical is responsible for regulating your level of tiredness. It helps signal to the rest of the body when it's time to sleep.

This is why people turn to coffee to get a quick jolt of energy when they start to feel tired or mentally rundown. By blocking adenosine production, caffeine can create a synthetic or artificially induced feeling of alertness and energy.

But as every coffee drinker knows, that energized feeling is all too often short lived. It's followed by an "energy crash" that can leave you feeling fatigued and desperately searching for another cup of joe.

However, what you may not realize is that the energy fix you get from coffee causes absolute chaos within the brain. Left unchecked, it can eventually cause the brain to turn on itself – becoming auto-cannibalistic – going into a state where it actually destroys vital components needed for healthy brain activity.

You expose your brain to serious health risks when you constantly try to "fool" it into thinking it has enough energy to function normally.

The Real Truth About Coffee

Coffee works to fool the brain in two major ways…

As mentioned earlier, it blocks the function of adenosine by interfering with the normal signals being sent to alert the body that it's time to sleep. When the brain doesn't receive the signals for sleep it recognizes something is wrong. The brain then sends out more receptors to search for more adenosine.

This means that once the caffeine from the coffee wears off, a higher amount of adenosine remains in action, beyond what the brain requires. A high concentration of adenosine in the brain prevents neuron receptors from functioning properly.

This eventually leads to what is sometimes called "brain fog". When in this state, you start to feel physically tired… mentally exhausted… and your thoughts become cloudy and difficult to process. It can be hard to concentrate or remember. Put plainly, you're too tired to think.

What you may not know is that this sudden energy crash jeopardizes the health of your brain in another way, too…

Once the coffee buzz wears off, the brain quickly realizes something's missing. It begins a desperate search to replace this key element that's responsible for keeping brain function running smoothly and your mind sharp and active.

So what is it that is actually missing from the brain?

It's a unique chemically based neurotransmitter called acetylcholine. This brain chemical has a direct role in the successful operation and function of all the cognitive activity inside the brain. If you've read this far, you've noticed that acetylcholine comes up again and again in connection with brain health.

It's responsible for controlling such things as attention span, sleep, intelligence, mood, arousal, and other basic functions. High levels of acetylcholine in the brain keep your mind clear and sharp. But when those levels are low, the results can be disastrous.

When the brain is deprived of acetylcholine, it goes on a frantic search to replenish its supply. Other brain chemicals are then released as "acetylcholine scavengers" and the most common place where they find this essential chemical is in the membranes of nerve cells.

Stripping acetylcholine from nerve cells will eventually damage brain health – hence the auto-cannibalistic effect mentioned earlier. The trillions of neurons in the brain require a steady supply of acetylcholine to sustain normal brain function.

When the coffee buzz wears off, the brain starts to tap into the stored reserves of acetylcholine in order to keep neurons functioning properly.

By constantly repeating this vicious cycle in which the brain has to tap into its reserves of acetylcholine, you drain those reserves and deprive the neurons of this essential neurotransmitter.

By stealing acetylcholine from nerve cells, the brain is essentially destroying any chance of maintaining healthy long-term brain activity. The nervous system can't work without sufficient amounts of acetylcholine. The communication between all areas of the brain will eventually slow down, leading to a greater risk of brain aging and a host of other problems.

Does Coffee Help Your Brain at All?

In spite of all this, moderate amounts of coffee or tea may have some health benefits. The truth of the matter is, coffee and the brain have a love-hate relationship.

Five Amazing Benefits of DMAE

Increasing the amount of DMAE in your diet or taking a DMAE supplement provides a variety of health benefits. This nutrient:

- Reduces symptoms associated with ADHD
- Enhances memory and brain power
- Reduces symptoms associated with both Alzheimer's and dementia
- Prevents depression
- Inhibits the appearance of wrinkles

Make sure you never let your brain go without a healthy supply of DMAE. Studies indicate that DMAE supplements are very safe and offer little risk of side effects if taken as directed. Be sure to speak with your doctor before adding this nutrient to your daily supplement intake.

Some studies suggest that drinking coffee in moderation may offer some positive benefits to brain health.

This research indicates that coffee could help lower your risk for general cognitive decline and even diseases like dementia and Alzheimer's. The reason is coffee's natural ability to prevent and reduce inflammation in the brain.

In a study published in the *Journal of Neuroscience*, Professor Gregory Freund and his team of researchers from the University of Illinois conducted an experiment to test the effects of caffeine on mice with hypoxia – a condition that causes cognitive and learning problems due to a reduction of oxygen in the body.

Creating a state of hypoxia in the mice caused a chain reaction in their brains. First, brain cells were triggered to release more of the brain chemical adenosine. This influx of adenosine activates caspase-1 enzymes, which in turn cause a higher production of cytokine IL-1ß – a known cause of inflammation.

Researchers tested to see if caffeine would help combat the dangerous effects of brain inflammation. What they found might shed some light on how to undo the effects of brain aging among people most at risk.

The mice in the test group given caffeine had a lower occurrence of inflammation and experienced a 33 percent faster memory recovery than the mice not given caffeine.

Researchers found the caffeine blocked all activity of the neurotransmitter adenosine and inhibited caspase-1-related inflammation. This type of inflammation plays a key role in many neurodegenerative diseases like Alzheimer's and dementia.

As a result there is some possible merit to consuming a moderate amount of coffee or other caffeinated beverages to protect the brain from inflammation-related health problems. The key to the successful balance is to avoid becoming dependent on caffeinated beverages, as too much caffeine can put you at greater risk of poor brain health.

What Should You Do?

The good news is that even if your brain has been suffering for years from the side effects caused by drinking too much caffeine – you can still repair the damage and improve brain function.

First, start by reducing the amount of coffee you consume on a daily basis. This will help put the natural balance back into your brain, so it starts to produce the right amount of critical brain chemicals like acetylcholine and adenosine.

Second, it's also important to give a sluggish brain the boost it needs to improve brain activity and keep your memory sharp – especially when your brain has been subjected to years and years of caffeine damage.

There are specific nutrients that can help get brain health back on track, allowing you to experience significant improvements and renewed cognitive abilities.

The next chapter will discuss these nutrients…

Chapter Eleven

Amazing Nutrients That Undo the Damage Coffee has Done to Your Brain

No matter how long you've been drinking coffee or other caffeine products, it's important to know that it's never too late to start repairing the damage.

You can easily strengthen the brain's defenses by providing the right nutrient support. Certain nutrients have been scientifically proven to naturally support better cognitive and mental health even after years of drinking coffee.

When it comes to helping the brain recover from caffeine wear and tear, the two most useful nutrients are choline and DMAE.

Choline

When it comes to improving memory and brain health, *choline is a must*. Without this nutrient, brain malfunction is almost unavoidable.

Recent studies have even revealed that a newborn must have an adequate supply of choline to enjoy healthy brain activity. As a result, pregnant and nursing mothers are encouraged to make sure they get enough choline in their diet.

Animal studies also prove this powerful nutrient can cause life-long changes to the structure and development of the brain – resulting in long-term memory-boosting benefits.

Choline is commonly linked to the vitamin B complex of nutrients because it works harmoniously together with B vitamins like folic acid (B9) and cobalamin (B12) to keep the brain, heart and other vital organs healthy.

The best evidence that choline is essential for healthy brain function is the fact that it's the main building block of acetylcholine, the vital neurotransmitter discussed in the previous chapter.

Under normal circumstances the brain is perfectly capable of producing healthy amounts of the brain chemicals it needs. But the brains of coffee drinkers may require a little extra help because caffeine interferes with the normal processes.

When the brain lacks enough choline, the symptoms are hard to ignore. It's common to experience both physical and mental symptoms of deficiency. These include. . .

- Difficulty sleeping

- Feeling distracted

- Foggy or cloudy thoughts

- Irritability

- Regular bouts of fatigue – both physical and mental

- Trouble maintaining balance

People who are lacking or flat out deficient in choline are more likely to have trouble remembering details. They may find it's a struggle to quickly grasp and process new information.

It's essential for good brain health to keep the brain supplied with choline.

More choline means you will have adequate levels of acetylcholine, and your memory and other cognitive faculties will be able to function at a higher level. There is plenty of research to show choline is a remarkable brain-saving nutrient…

In one study conducted at Northwestern University in Chicago, researchers looked at the general effects of choline on the brain. Participants were given a series of memory tests at the beginning of the study. All the participants scored below average on these tests, indicating they were suffering from choline deficiency.

Next, participants were divided into two groups. One group received extra choline for the duration of 24 weeks while the other group did not. At the end of the period, researchers repeated the same memory tests.

What were the results?

The group that did not receive added choline did not experience any changes or score higher on their memory tests. However, the test results from the

Metals and Minerals Found in the Body

Below is a list of 24 of the most common potentially toxic metals or minerals found in the environment. Trace amounts of them can be found in the blood or body tissues of most people in developed countries.

Some of them are needed in small amounts for good health, such as copper, selenium, chromium, manganese, vanadium and zinc. But excessively high levels of even these necessary metals can be toxic.

Others, such as antimony, arsenic, lead, mercury and cadmium, are toxic to the body in ANY amount and should be avoided entirely. Iron is needed by the body in fairly large amounts, but is toxic above those levels.

If your level of any one of these metals becomes too high, it can put your brain at risk for neurodegeneration, cognitive decline, Alzheimer's and dementia… and a host of other serious health problems:

• Antimony	• Manganese
• Arsenic	• Mercury
• Bismuth	• Nickel
• Cadmium	• Platinum
• Cerium	• Selenium
• Chromium	• Silver
• Cobalt	• Tellurium
• Copper	• Thallium
• Gallium	• Tin
• Gold	• Uranium
• Iron	• Vanadium
• Lead	• Zinc

http://www.lef.org/protocols/health_concerns/heavy_metal_detoxification_01.htm

second group proved to be drastically different.

Researchers found participants in the choline group experienced a dramatic improvement in memory function. In fact, they passed all their memory tests with ease and scored well above average.

Further research into the brain-saving benefits of choline have scientists pushing for more tests to determine if choline could actually be the solution to preventing – and even treating – brain diseases like Parkinson's and Alzheimer's.

This line of research is very promising because even now, studies reveal the brains of most people with Alzheimer's disease have low levels of acetylcholine. Clearly then the relationship between this brain chemical and disease prevention is strong.

You need to make sure your brain is getting a therapeutically effective amount of choline to lower your risk for memory problems and diseases.

A balanced diet is one way to increase the amount of choline in the brain. Eating foods containing lecithin – available as a supplement or a food additive – can help deliver a daily supply of choline to the brain.

The body breaks down lecithin and is able to naturally convert it into choline. Lecithin is used to help bind fat from foods to water. That's why it's added to foods like ice cream, chocolate bars and mayonnaise.

The body converts lecithin into choline, which can be readily absorbed into the brain and used to produce acetylcholine.

For the average person, a daily choline intake of 425 milligrams (women) or 550 milligrams (men) will prevent deficiency. Adding lecithin-rich foods to your diet helps achieve a healthy level of acetylcholine safely and naturally. Some examples are. . .

- Cabbage
- Cauliflower
- Chickpeas
- Eggs
- Green beans
- Lentils
- Liver
- Red Meat
- Rice

- Soy lecithin

- Soybeans

- Split peas

In addition to harming your brain and increasing your risk of memory-related problems, a lack of choline can also put you at greater risk for atherosclerosis and liver disease. So making sure there's enough choline in your diet benefits your health in multiple ways.

DMAE (2-Dimethylaminoethanol)

The second organic compound that supports the body's production of acetylcholine is known as DMAE or 2-dimethylaminoethanol. In small amounts, DMAE occurs naturally throughout the brain.

DMAE is one of the building blocks for choline. Both of these nutrients work hand in hand to give the brain a chance to reach maximum memory and learning capacity.

When the brain's DMAE levels are adequate, memory and overall brain function dramatically improve. A number of studies conducted on DMAE prove that it helps:

- Improve memory

- Enhance learning capabilities

- Boost brain circulation

- Promote healthier blood oxygen levels

- Strengthen the integrity of brain cells

What makes DMAE such a unique nutrient is that it enhances your cognitive ability and increases your overall level of mental energy, too. This nutrient is able to cross the blood-brain barrier quickly and be absorbed into the brain. The blood-brain barrier screens out many substances – usually those that aren't healthy for the brain, but occasionally some healthy nutrients as well.

So eating foods or taking supplements rich in DMAE is important if you want to enjoy maximum brain health.

According to one study published in *Nature,* a pound of selected seafoods contains a few milligrams of DMAE that can be easily utilized by the brain.

There are three kinds of fish that are naturally rich in DMAE:

- Salmon

- Anchovies

- Sardines or pilchards

Many Mediterranean dishes call for these fish in their recipes. They can be a tasty and fun way to increase your DMAE levels.

A daily DMAE supplement can also improve brain health…

One published study evaluated a group of 80 participants to determine the benefits of DMAE on the brain. The evaluations revealed that those supplementing with DMAE experienced better mental activity and felt much more alert than those not taking the supplement.

DMAE works wonders in refueling the brain and preventing depletion of both choline and acetylcholine.

This nutrient also helps the brain sustain adequate energy levels to prevent brain decay and age-related cognitive decline. This sort of nutrient-based energy is much more effective than synthetic alternatives like caffeine that end up doing more harm to the brain than good.

Let Go of the Cup of Joe

The combined effects of choline and DMAE can help the brain recover from the chaos caused by coffee and other caffeinated drinks.

As time goes by, once you reduce the amount of coffee you drink – or even eliminate it all together – don't go back to relying on it when you need energy or you're experiencing brain fog.

Instead, make use of natural, safe energy boosters that won't jeopardize your brain or reduce your cognitive ability.

RESOURCES AND FURTHER READING:

http://www.livestrong.com/article/251172-benefits-to-the-brain-from-choline/#ixzz2BO5bDsXE

http://www.vitaminstuff.com/choline.html

http://hc.alsearsmd.com/ct/26090135:6512321030:m:1:466481828:DE4846BD2F60DD8752A567BD6D06FC3D:r

http://www.nutraingredients.com/Research/Caffeine-may-block-brain-inflammation-to-reduce-dementia-risk

http://www.livestrong.com/article/458485-foods-containing-dmae/#ixzz2C1U23MGn

http://www.brainpower.org/research/dmae.html

Chapter Twelve

Environmental Toxins That Attack Your Brain

Toxins constantly attack your body every day. They are in the air you breathe… the foods you eat… the water you drink, and a variety of products you use every day and probably don't even think about – shampoos, cleaners and other household products, even clothing and mattresses, or the material used to build your house or the building where you work.

The immune system has the job of first identifying toxic elements and foreign invaders, and then fighting them off and safely removing them from your body before they damage your health.

Under normal circumstances, the immune system rises to the challenge and faces these toxic invaders head on – being the clear victor most of the time. Typical examples are microbes and parasites, or cancer cells (which form in a healthy body all the time, even though few people know it.)

However, there are situations when certain environmental toxins can slip past your immune system's defenses and subtly begin an all out assault on your brain.

This proves to be the case with many metals, especially those classified as heavy metals…

Not all heavy metals are bad. Some are healthy nutrients. Your body needs them because they play an important role in specific bodily functions. For example, zinc is an essential nutrient to improve memory and overall cognitive health, but it's also classified as a heavy metal.

Another example is the metal lithium (usually classified as a "light" metal). Certain medical treatments require lithium to manage various health disorders. However, if levels of lithium in the blood become too high, serious toxicity can result. Chromium, a heavy metal, is likewise essential in small amounts but toxic in large amounts.

When it comes to these substances, balance is critical. If levels are too high, the metals can't be properly excreted. As a result, toxic amounts build up in the body's tissues, including the brain.

Heavy metals make the top of the list of toxic substances that can destroy brain function. Studies show heavy metal toxicity is detrimental on both a short-term and long-term scale, resulting in severe damage to nerve and brain function. These in turn affect every other system and function in your body.

The key to combating the negative side effects of heavy metal exposure is to be aware of the symptoms and be able to spot them at their earliest stages. Know how heavy metals can enter into your body so you can lower your risk of excessive exposure.

General symptoms associated with brain and nervous system heavy metal toxicity include:

• Fatigue

• Hearing, vision or taste changes

• Impaired memory

• Irritability

• Muscle weakness

• Myoclonus (twitching muscles)

• Nervousness

• Numbness and tingling

• Personality changes

• Seizures

• Tremors

• Trouble concentrating

Many average household items contain toxic metals or chemicals that can threaten brain function. It's important to become aware of the ways you might be coming into contact with certain toxic metals without knowing it.

Here are a few examples of how metals can make their way into your body and alter brain activity:

• **Cosmetics** – Beauty products contain various chemicals. But it might surprise you to know that the Food and Drug Administration (FDA) allows small amounts of the heavy metal mercury to be used in certain types of eye make-up as a preservative. In fact, during the mid-1990s several individuals using a cosmetic product manufactured in Mexico suffered mercury poisoning.

• **Household items that contain mercury** – Besides cosmetics, traces of mercury can also be found in fluorescent light bulbs, blood pressure devices, and thermostats. These devices are generally safe as long as the glass containing the mercury is not broken. But breakage can result in the release of a large amount of mercury.

- **Plumbing pipes** – Water pipes that were installed more than 90 years ago pose a risk of lead exposure, including those in municipal water systems in older cities. Lead poisoning is probably one of the most well known forms of heavy metal poisoning. It has disastrous effects on brain health. Lead can easily accumulate in the brain, causing serious damage to the neurons responsible for your learning and memory abilities.

- **Aluminum overload:** Antacids, cosmetics, cookware, and pain relievers can all increase your risk for aluminum exposure. There's no conclusive evidence that high levels of aluminum damage the brain, but there's also no evidence to suggest it offers any health benefits. Studies show aluminum has no natural function in the human body. The prudent thing to do is avoid it. Some studies have reported that high amounts of aluminum was been found in the brains of people suffering from Alzheimer's disease and dementia, but other studies contradict these findings. More evidence is needed before it is known whether the metal causes these conditions.

> ## Ten Foods Proven to Reduce Inflammation
>
> Reducing the frequency of inflammation flare-ups can be safely done by including foods with natural anti-inflammatory agents in your daily diet.
>
> Here are ten delicious foods that have been scientifically proven to combat inflammation and promote better health:
>
> - Blueberries
> - Broccoli
> - Cherries (tart)
> - Fish
> - Green tea
> - Kelp
> - Nuts
> - Olive oil
> - Papaya
> - Turmeric (Curcumin)
>
> Making these foods a regular feature in your daily diet not only calms fiery inflammation, but can also reduce your need for prescription or over-the-counter painkillers that cause serious damage to your health when used long-term. Pain-killing drugs should be used only sparingly and on a temporary basis, to get over episodes of acute pain. They are not safe for long-term use.
>
> http://www.losethebackpain.com/blog/2012/03/12/foods-that-fight-inflammation/

Paying attention to your risk of exposure to heavy metals and other environmental toxins will lower your risk for cognitive impairments and prevent over all brain health from being jeopardized.

If you want to get rid of excessive metals in your body, seek the help of a naturopathic doctor (N.D.) or an integrative M.D. who is receptive to alternative medicine. Ask them to give you a test to measure your levels of various metals – and about chelation, the best remedy for removing these metals from your body.

ADDITIONAL READING:

http://www.bidmc.org/YourHealth/HolisticHealth/MentalHealth.aspx?ChunkID=14255

Epilogue

It's Never Too Late to Protect Your Brain

If you've read this far, you now know there are many different ways to protect your precious brain!

Maintaining the basics is a must and should never be overlooked. Basic requirements like a healthy diet… regular physical and mental exercise… and adequate nutrient supplementation provide both short-term and long-term benefits to your brain.

It's just as important to make an effort to eliminate risk factors associated with brain atrophy and disease. Doing this gives your brain a fighting chance to prevent further damage caused by free radicals, toxins, and other outside factors and to repair the damage they've already done.

As more research sheds light on various hazards to brain health, it's critical you make it a priority to reduce your exposure to new risk factors as they become known.

Do whatever you can to nourish your mind and create the perfect environment for it!

The preceding chapters have given you the knowledge you need to successfully keep your mind supercharged with the fuel it needs to function at its peak level. Try as many of these tips as you can, and it's extremely likely your cognitive abilities will improve and you'll soon find you can tackle whatever challenges come your way. You'll enjoy a clear, quick, energetic and active mind.

Diseases like dementia and Alzheimer's will become less and less of a threat as you patiently find ways to lower your exposure to the risk factors associated with these diseases.

Follow this report's guidelines and tips for the long run and you'll preserve the health of your neurons and other brain cells. Your priceless neurotransmitters like acetylcholine and serotonin will keep the communications network in your brain working at lightning-fast speeds and peak efficiency.

This is a good place to mention that foods and supplements work their magic over the long term. Plan to eat right and take brain-supporting supplements for the rest of your life, and don't expect to see results in mere days or weeks – although that can happen – especially in people who are extremely deficient in vital nutrients. They can experience remarkable turnarounds very fast.

But even though some people do get quick relief, supplements aren't like pharmaceutical drugs. You don't take two and feel better in the morning. The benefits are felt over the course of months and even years.

The most important thing to remember is this: Getting older does not mean you have to accept losing your mind. If you pay attention to the needs of your brain right now you can stay mentally sharp… focused… and constantly active no matter how many years go by!